PRAISE FOR
THE FIVE BLESSINGS OF IFÁ

"It's about time for more books like these to be written. Gabrielle does something special by weaving Isese Ifá and its diasporic variations into one cohesive voice of knowledge. No matter where on Earth you come from, Gabrielle ensures you'll see a part of yourself through her text. This book is one part study, two parts soul, and that's why it'll be a book to reach for even long after we're gone."

> —EHIME ORA, author of *Ancestors Said* and *Spirits Come from Water*

"An indispensable read that integrates Afro-Indigenous spirituality into contemporary environmental discussions."

> —JESSICA HERNANDEZ, PhD, author of *Fresh Banana Leaves* and *Growing Papaya Trees*

"A must-read for anyone who is diasporic and trying to find tools for nurturing a future on occupied Indigenous land alongside Black life and culture. . . . With deep examination and knowledge, Felder seeks and finds the five blessings of Ifá not in the mythical past or tradition, but in real history and in the present—in the very places where future dreaming work can occur. I walked away from the book feeling renewed about the inventiveness of diasporic life, queer life, and Black life. Read this book if you like to dream with your friends!"

> —ALICE SPARKLY KAT, author of *Postcolonial Astrology*

"A spiritual homecoming. . . . Felder gives us coordinates of hope and survival, reminding us that the ancestors have much to show us about how to survive and how to brave the new world. As she writes, 'Growth is only possible if we look forward toward the future—and bring with us the tools of the past, like Ifá.' The future is awaiting the promise of our wisdom, and this book shows us how to fuse the technologies of the past so we may be better equipped for all that's to come. I loved reading this book; these are necessary materials to build the utopia we all deserve."

> —FARIHA RÓISÍN, author of *Who Is Wellness For?*, *How to Cure a Ghost*, and *Survival Takes a Wild Imagination*

". . . [Felder's] enthusiasm for 'the beauty and complexity of Black life and culture' is unfailingly enthusiastic and expansive."

THE FIVE
BLESSINGS
OF IFÁ

THE FIVE BLESSINGS OF IFÁ

RECLAIMING BLACK FUTURES THROUGH AFRO-INDIGENOUS SPIRITUALITY

GABRIELLE FELDER

North Atlantic Books
Huichin, unceded Ohlone land
Berkeley, California

North Atlantic Books
Huichin, unceded Ohlone land
2526 Martin Luther King Jr Way
Berkeley, CA 94704 USA
www.northatlanticbooks.com

Cover art © S_Chanjai246 via Shutterstock
and BBM via Alamy Stock Photo
Cover design by Jess Morphew
Book design by Happenstance Type-O-Rama

Printed in the United States of America

The Five Blessings of Ifá: Reclaiming Black Futures Through Afro-Indigenous Spirituality is sponsored and published by North Atlantic Books, an educational nonprofit that collaborates with partners to develop cross-cultural perspectives; nurture holistic views of art, science, the humanities, and healing; and seed personal and global transformation by publishing work on the relationship of body, spirit, and nature.

North Atlantic Books's publications are distributed to the US trade and internationally by Penguin Random House Publisher Services. For further information, visit our website at www.northatlanticbooks.com.

The authorized representative in the EU for product safety and compliance is Eucomply OÜ, Pärnu mnt 139b-14, 11317 Tallinn, Estonia, hello@eucompliancepartner.com, +33757690241.

Library of Congress Cataloging-in-Publication Data

Names: Felder, Gabrielle author
Title: The five blessings of Ifá : reclaiming Black futures through
    Afro-Indigenous spirituality / Gabrielle Felder.
Description: Huichin, unceded Ohlone land, Berkeley, California : North
    Atlantic Books, [2025] | Includes biographical information. | Includes
    bibliographical references and index. | Summary: "A guide to Black
    resistance, resilience, and healing, using the principles of the West
    African spiritual tradition of Ifá." -- Provided by publisher.
Identifiers: LCCN 2025016515 (print) | LCCN 2025016516 (ebook) | ISBN
    9798889841043 paperback | ISBN 9798889841036 ebook
Subjects: LCSH: Ifa | African Americans--Religion
Classification: LCC BL2532.I33 F45 2025 (print) | LCC BL2532.I33 (ebook)
LC record available at https://lccn.loc.gov/2025016515
LC ebook record available at https://lccn.loc.gov/2025016516

1 2 3 4 5 6 7 8 9 KPC 30 29 28 27 26 25

*In loving memory of my grandmother
Ida Louise Scott, whose stories, recipes,
and love live on in this book and through me.*

CONTENTS

INTRODUCTION:
Good and Evil

Since I was a young child, I wanted to learn about the secrets hidden in nature. When I was in kindergarten, my teacher taught a lesson on the plant life cycle. She taught us how to germinate seeds with a wet cotton ball inside a Ziploc bag that she taped to our classroom window. Watching the seedling germinate awakened an insatiable curiosity within me. I replicated the classroom experiment at home on my own several times, each time developing a deeper and deeper appreciation for nature and the art of experimentation.

I jumped at the opportunity to learn more about the world around me. My adolescent years were spent at museums, science centers, and aquariums. I felt at home in tactile learning environments where I could interact with the world outside the classroom. I was fortunate enough to go on two outdoor science field trips with my school when I was in sixth and seventh grade. In sixth grade, my school spent a week in the Southern California mountains as part of our outdoor education program. Aside from playing in my backyard or at the park, I didn't spend time in nature growing up. My school field trip was my first opportunity to spend an extended period of time deep in the forest. After spending a week picking blackberries, collecting quartz crystals, and hiking through the mountains, my eyes were opened to the wonder of nature on a large scale. While my childhood seed germination experiment showed me the intricacy of life, outdoor education showed me the vastness and interconnectedness of the world.

My fascination with a kindergarten classroom activity grew into a life-long career studying science and technology. I wanted to understand the origin of everything. I wanted to unlock the secrets to the seeds of life and figure out how something so small could grow into something of incomprehensible magnitude. I became an evolutionary scientist, studying both ecology and anthropology in undergrad. Studying evolutionary ecology and anthropology brought me closer to understanding the origins of life on earth. According to evolutionary biology, there are three main domains that represent all life on earth: Bacteria, Archaea, and Eukarya. The relationship among these domains is often represented by a phylogenetic tree, a diagram that shows the biological relationship between organisms. In the universal phylogenetic tree, each of the three domains branch off into smaller and smaller branches, representing connections through shared ancestry.

Spiritual traditions all over the world attempt to uncover the root or seed of the universal phylogenetic tree as they seek to explain the origin of life and the creation of the universe. Ifá turns to nature to seek the answers to the universal secrets that birthed the cosmos. Ifá represents the wisdom, power, and potential of seeds. All of nature is sacred within Ifá, but seeds hold the most significance.

The seeds from the sacred palm tree are called *ikin* and they represent the power of Ọ̀rúnmìlà, the *orisa* of wisdom and divination. In the Yoruba creation myth, Ọ̀rúnmìlà is one of the few orisas present when the universe was created, earning him the title ẹlẹ́rìí ìpín, the witness to creation. The sacred palm tree is regarded as the tree of life, and the ikin represent the seeds of all creation. Ikin are one of the most sacred objects an *aborisa*, devotee of Ifá, can receive. Not all palm nuts are considered sacred; only palm nuts with four or more "eyes" are used in Ifá. Through the eyes of the palm nuts, Ọ̀rúnmìlà is able to divine by "seeing" all the possibilities that exist.

In many ways, Ifá is the seed of the African diaspora. Ifá's cultural impact affects every aspect of Black life. It can be felt through the spiritual traditions, food, music, and relationships Black people create across the diaspora. Just as enslaved Africans braided seeds into their hair to carry to the New World, Ifá was carried across the Atlantic, woven in the cultural and spiritual fabric of West Africa. Like a seed, Ifá took root in the Americas, growing and evolving into diverse cultural customs. The different branches or variations of Ifá can be found in the United States, Cuba, Brazil, Haiti, and beyond.

When I began writing this book, my plan was to keep it from my family for as long as possible. My relationship with my family is complicated by our differing religious beliefs, upbringing, and politics. The world my parents portrayed was one filled with good and evil. Everything in the universe fell into one of those two categories. God, church, school, and family were good. Essentially everything else was bad. As a queer child struggling to come to terms with my sexuality and gender identity, I grew up in fear of myself, my parents, and my family. Though my parents had portrayed family as a haven from the outside world, my queerness made me feel ostracized, and I quickly learned it was best to keep to myself. A lot of the fear my parents instilled in me was rooted in their religious beliefs. Most of the conversations I remember having with my mom about Christianity centered on the concept of hell. My mom would wait until we were trapped in the car together on a long car ride to warn me about the fire and brimstone that awaited me in death if I chose to forsake her religion. The imagery she conjured was made to invoke fear within me and to scare me into obedience. Even as a young child, I knew I didn't want to make all my life decisions based on fear.

Over time, I grew skeptical of my parents' and grandparents' religion. I struggled to feel connected in church and often wondered if I was missing something. As my love for science grew, it became harder and harder to reconcile what I was learning in school with what I was learning in the Bible. I felt a deep connection to the world around me and was convinced that the secrets of the universe would be revealed to me through nature and ancient languages.

My spiritual journey began in high school. Growing up, I was fortunate enough to have friends from different cultural and religious backgrounds. These friendships introduced me to new ways of seeing the world that were different than the ones I was taught growing up. In high school, I would spend hours contemplating the universe and discussing spiritual philosophy with a close friend. Through our conversations, she taught me about the Hindu understanding of the universe as an interconnected web of creation. We read Siddhartha together and went down Wikipedia rabbit holes reading about different sects of Buddhism.

I was introduced to African diasporic spirituality in college. For my birthday, one of my best friends bought me a book about Louisiana voodoo and a book about New Age witchcraft. The book on New Age witchcraft was full of "practical magic," spells and rituals that used easily accessible ingredients that could be found in your local grocery store or in your own backyard. Love spells, spells for success, and spells for self-confidence and inner peace were made accessible through this book. Using herbs like rosemary and mint, rose petals, honey, and a few crystals, suddenly I could manifest all my heart's desires. I had fun playing around with some of the spells, and I slowly began to grow my collection of witchy books. Though I was reluctant to admit it, I was drawn to any spell that claimed to attract love. My college years were spent navigating the predominantly white spaces within academia, leaving me feeling isolated and unsure of myself and my relationships. I desperately looked for ways to cultivate a sense of love and belonging.

Over time, I began to mix love spells from my New Age witchcraft books with the ones I found in my voodoo books. At the time, voodoo's mysterious and seemingly dark nature intrigued and intimidated me. I'd always figured that I had some distant familial connection to Louisiana voodoo since my grandmother's family was originally from Louisiana. I enjoyed incorporating spells and rituals from a place I had an ancestral connection to. While I was home on summer break, when I was sure my parents weren't around, I'd flip through the book, paying special attention to spells and perfumes that promised to strengthen love and attraction, increase self-confidence, and cut soul ties and other toxic connections. Using roses and oranges from my parents' garden, I attempted to make perfume oils inspired by recipes developed by Marie Leveau, the queen of Louisiana voodoo. Something about collecting the roses and oranges from my own backyard unlocked something in me. Suddenly, I was transported back to my childhood, when I imagined my backyard as an enchanted forest where fairies and other magical beings lived. With childlike eyes, I was beginning to appreciate the magic and beauty around me while rediscovering the usefulness of the herbs, fruits, and vegetables I often took for granted.

Throughout college and into graduate school, I continued to collect books on New Age and Black American spiritual practices. While I lived in Seattle, I visited an occult shop in my neighborhood where I stocked up on perfume oils that promised me luck and love, votive candles in glass jars decorated in honor of the orisa Ọṣun, and books about Black and African spiritual practices. As I began researching the differences between hoodoo and voodoo, I realized how much depth and nuance there was within the realm of Black spiritual traditions. Slowly, I began to lose interest in New Age spirituality, which I began to view more and more as profit-driven and superficial. New Age rituals tended to be very object-based and required a slew of bowls, crystals, herbs, and candles for every spell. Witch kits composed of white sage, incense, crystals, and tarot cards sold for over $100 on websites like Etsy and Urban Outfitters. The more I studied hoodoo, the more I realized how much New Age spiritual traditions were appropriated from Indigenous, Black, and Asian practices.

While both hoodoo and New Age rituals incorporated elements from Indigenous American traditions, the relationship between hoodoo and Indigenous wisdom felt more authentic. As a Black American tradition, hoodoo's incorporation of Indigenous American wisdom grew out of cultural exchange among Black and Indigenous people living in the Southern United States. Many of the traditions were rooted in an understanding of Southern American herbalism, which incorporated both African and Indigenous American plant knowledge. I slowly began to shift my focus to primarily Black American folk traditions like hoodoo and voodoo. I wanted to focus on practices that had cultural relevance and meaning to me. Studying these traditions was a path toward reclaiming my heritage and discovering lost traditions that my family attempted to bury and hide. As a descendant of enslaved Africans and a child raised by evangelical parents, there was never any conversation about more traditional African and African American spiritual practices. Folksy traditions and superstitions colored my childhood. Cooking black-eyed peas and collard greens on New Year's Day attracted wealth and prosperity. Sweeping someone's feet could send them to jail. Through the study of hoodoo and voodoo, I realized those superstitions were rooted in Black and African spiritual practices. Whether my family realized it or not, African spiritual traditions continued to shape and influence their lives.

In 2020, after studying Black American folk traditions for a few years, I began to study Ifá. Over the years, I pored over several books that explained the rituals and practices of hoodoo and voodoo. I read about honey jars used to draw and attract love and luck. I learned which passages from Psalms I could use to protect against enemies. I felt like I had learned virtually everything I could learn from scouring the internet. After writing a post about hoodoo traditions and spells on Instagram, I received a very strongly worded comment from someone who essentially told me that I had a lot to learn. Instead of taking offense at their comment, I was intrigued. I had reached a block in my research, and I was eager to find new channels for information. We ended up exchanging phone numbers, and on that call they introduced me to several hoodoo practitioners who ran various closed groups. I joined a few groups and learned the basics of making spiritual baths, listened to some popular Black spiritual podcasts, and discovered new books from Black hoodoo traditionalists. I consumed everything Zora Neale Hurston wrote, foraged for herbs, and bought candles at Indigenous-owned spiritual shops. Quickly, my interest in Black modalities of healing blossomed into an obsession. I was inspired by Zora's immersive anthropological approach to life. Throughout her life, Zora was initiated into several different secret societies and spiritual traditions in the United States, Jamaica, and Haiti. I admired her approach and dedication to experimentation. Reading books about Black spiritual traditions could only take me so far. I wanted not just to read about different Afro-diasporic traditions, but to practice them.

After listening to *A Little Juju Podcast,* I impulsively booked a two-hour Ifá reading through an *ilé* I had never heard of. An ilé is a spiritual house or community within the tradition of Ifá. They essentially function as spiritual centers, not dissimilar to churches, that are typically headed by a *babalawo* or *iyanifa,* the priests and priestesses within the tradition. I'd combed the internet for hours, searching for babalawos in Portland, Oregon, where I was living at the time. Finding a Black babalawo in Portland proved a nearly impossible feat, so I expanded my search, hoping to find someone that provided services online. At the time, I knew very little about Ifá other than that it was a tradition from Nigeria that involved the worship of orisas, the gods and goddesses within the tradition.

The reading took place deep in the COVID-19 pandemic one afternoon over video call. I was greeted by a middle-aged Black man with a kind face. He introduced himself as Chief Awósanmí Sékou Alájé, a babalawo who trained in both Cuba and Nigeria and had years of experience that took him around the world. He explained that his ilé was based in Brooklyn, New York, but he offered spiritual services to people across the United States. After asking me for some basic information, he began the reading. I watched intently as he swung the *opele*, or divination chain, on a circular wooden board. The reading concluded with Chief Alájé explaining the recommendations he gleaned through the divination process. I took diligent notes on everything he said, eager to absorb as much information from the experience as possible. That reading would launch me into a years-long journey to better understand the mysteries of Ifá and to better understand myself.

After a camping trip with my partner in the mountains of Oregon, where I saw the Milky Way Galaxy for the first time, I decided that I would begin my Ifá apprenticeship under Chief Awósanmí Sékou Alájé. Chief Alájé's ilé focuses on Isese, a traditional form of Ifá closely connected to spiritual teachers and lineages in Nigeria. Sitting under the stars, it felt like the right time for me to move past fear and explore the unknown. Training as an *ọmọ awo*, a "child of mysteries" or apprentice, meant hours spent studying *odu*, the foundational spiritual concepts of Ifá in the form of symbolism and sacred poetry. I learned songs and practiced reciting prayers in Yoruba, a language that was completely unfamiliar to me. I was assigned an iyanifa to provide me with more one-on-one lessons. With her guidance I sped through the online and virtual lessons and was finally ready to receive my own Ifá shrine. In Ifá, receiving your own shrine, also known as receiving your Hand of Ifá or Isefa, is a huge step that symbolizes the beginning of your journey. The process requires specific divinations and rituals that ultimately culminate in a naming ceremony where you receive your Ifá name. After I received my Hand of Ifá, I became an aborisa, or devotee of the orisa. This process symbolizes your dedication to Ifá and is the first step toward initiation should you choose to go down that path.

The year my Ifá journey began was full of personal and political turmoil. I graduated from a challenging and mentally draining graduate school program shortly after the murder of George Floyd. I was living in Portland, Oregon, and I felt paralyzed by the political uproar happening just outside my door. My mental health was in shambles after graduate school, and combined with the COVID pandemic, I felt overwhelming feelings of anxiety, paranoia, and dread. Unable to leave my house, I buried myself in books, reading as much as I could about the historical forces behind white supremacy and racial inequality in the United States and around the world. I studied the work of Frank B. Wilderson III, Frantz Fanon, Saidiya Hartman, and other Black radical scholars. I studied Indigenous American traditions and Eastern religions and compared their core beliefs to those found within Ifá and other African traditional religions. I discovered the interconnectedness of Black political movements and Black African spirituality as well as the similarities between African, Indigenous, Hindu, and Buddhist cosmology.

It was clear to me that whether we knew it or not, African spiritual traditions guide and inform so much of Black life. These traditions have served as both a guide on our path toward liberation and a means of cross-cultural connection. Countless examples from across the diaspora illustrate the unique syncretization of African, Indigenous American, and Christian beliefs that created cultural and spiritual traditions unique to the Caribbean, Latin America, and the United States. Ifá, herbalism, and community gardening were grounding forces for me during one of the most mentally and emotionally challenging periods in my life. My time spent making *ose*, a weekly ritual that focuses on tending to your personal shrines, served as a meditative practice that forced me to slow down and take stock of how I was doing emotionally and mentally. The set routine of making ose provided me with structure and a space to voice my concerns out loud while grounding me in nature and ancestral wisdom.

Black people in the diaspora have incorporated African values into our lives and allowed them to shape how we related to each other and the world around us. We've formed families, built communities, formed cross-cultural coalitions, and overcome adversity using African values as our foundational and guiding force.

THE ROOTS OF IFÁ

Ifá is a ten-thousand-year-old spiritual tradition from the Yoruba people who reside in modern-day Nigeria and Benin. During the transatlantic slave trade, Ifá, along with other West and Central African traditions, was carried across the ocean. The most popular and best-known orisas were carried to the Americas. Ọṣun (Oshun), Esu (Elégbà, Papa Legba, Elegua), Ṣàngó (Chango), Ọ̀rúnmìlà, Ọya, Yemayá, and Ògún are among the most popular and well-recognized orisas across the diaspora. European cultural and linguistic influence transformed Ifá into several well-known traditions through the diaspora, including Candomblé, Santería, and Lukumi. Traditional Yoruba dress mixed with Spanish and Portuguese colonial attire, Christian iconography replaced Yoruba depictions of the orisa, and Yoruba words became Hispanicized. Despite the inevitable changes that colonization brought to African diasporic cultures, the core traditions and beliefs within Ifá and its offshoots remains.

In Ifá, nature is viewed as the manifestation of Olódùmarè, the divine creator. The life force that runs throughout nature and the universe is known as *asé* (also spelled ashe or axe). Asé flows through all things, both living and nonliving. Asé provides practitioners with the power to actualize or manifest their blessing. In addition to asé, the orisas serve as another source of power within Ifá. The orisas (also spelled orishas or orichas) are the gods and goddesses of the tradition, the embodiment of forces of nature and concepts that have the power to influence human endeavors. They represent the many aspects of Olódùmarè.[1] There are thousands of orisas, with some specifically worshiped within the confines of a region or city.

The word *orisa* comes from the root word *orí*, meaning "spiritual head" in Yoruba. An orí can be thought of as one's consciousness. In Ifá, your orí is your sacred center that connects you to the rest of the world around you. An orisa is essentially an "elevated head" or an orí with unlimited potential. By passing through different stages of development, one's orí has the potential to reach that of an orisa. In fact, many of the Yoruba myths that surround the orisa are stories of ordinary people who, through incredible feats, became defied and ascended to the level of orisa. This concept that godliness lives in each of us is a central component to Ifá. By studying the orisas, Ifá practitioners seek to maintain balance within themselves, known as *iwa pele,* so that they may eventually reach a state of enlightenment.

The tradition employs a traditional divination technique called Ifá *didá* that uses one of the world's first binary systems to divulge information from the universe. In a way, Ifá can be thought of as a computer, using binary code to translate information downloaded from nature. An Ifá didá is traditionally performed by a babalawo or iyanifa. Initiation is a sacred ceremony that serves as a spiritual promotion of sorts. Ọmọ awos, students or apprentices of babalawos and iyanifas, undergo initiation after years of study and apprenticeship under the guidance of elders in their ilé, spiritual community. Initiation is not the final step or "goal" for ọmọ awos, but rather the beginning of a lifelong journey to learn the secrets of Ifá and master spiritual rituals. Babalawos and iyanifas are expected to dedicate their lives to the community, serving as spiritual leaders, teachers, and community builders. Initiation is not something to rush into or to take lightly. Depending on the traditions of your ilé, initiation ceremonies can require trips to Nigeria or Cuba, making the cost to initiate a huge barrier for some. The level of dedication required after initiating into the tradition can also be prohibitive for some. Both the cost and dedication required mean that initiation is not for everyone. Some people initiate into the tradition after a year of study, while others take five or more years to initiate. While some people are encouraged to initiate based on messages received during divination, for most initiation is a personal decision. For me, initiation isn't a priority for me due to the commitment both financially and spiritually to initiate fully into the tradition. There is a wealth of knowledge still to be learned as an aborisa.

During an Ifá didá, the babalawo, literally translated to "father of mysteries," uses sixteen sacred palm nuts to communicate with key orisas. Based on how the palm nuts fall, the babalawo or iyanifa, mother of Ifá, marks the *opón ifá,* the sacred divination tray, creating a unique pattern that corresponds to an odu, or divination. *Ebo,* sacrifice or offerings, are performed or given to ensure that the client has a "clear path" to access their blessings.

Blessing in Ifá center around five main components: Ire Àìkú, blessings of longevity; Ire Àjé, blessing of wealth and prosperity; Ire Ọkọ/Aya, blessings of marriage and partnership; Ire Ọmọ, blessings of children; and Ire Ìṣẹ́gun, blessing of victory over negative forces. The blessing of Àìkú or longevity is the most important, followed by the blessing of wealth, and so on. To live a fulfilled life according to Ifá is to live a long life surrounded by friends and family and to have an abundance of support to allow you to triumph during difficult times.

As I studied the practices within Ifá, I quickly realized that to truly grasp the intricacies of the tradition, I would need to learn Yoruba. Fluency isn't required, but an understanding of the language and the literal translations of the words is crucial. Colonialism uses language as a tool to shape one's worldview into that of their oppressors. When we translate from indigenous languages to English or Spanish or French, we lose important aspects of what our ancestors were trying to convey.

OTHER AFRICAN TRADITIONAL RELIGIONS

Ifá is just one of many traditions that were carried with enslaved Africans across the Atlantic Ocean. African traditional religions (ATRs) refer to the indigenous religions of African people across the continent and throughout the diaspora. ATRs share many similarities with other indigenous and non-Abrahamic religious traditions. Like other indigenous religions, ATRs are oral traditions, passed down through multigenerational storytelling, often involving sacred rites of passage before specific knowledge can be shared. The foundational basis of ATRs is a deep understanding and appreciation of nature in its fullness, which emphasizes the interconnectedness of humans, the natural landscape, climate, flora, fauna, and the cosmos. Most ATRs are technically polytheistic, though typically the multiple gods and goddesses within the tradition represent different aspects of the creator.

Contrary to popular belief, ATRs are dynamic traditions that are constantly changing. Divination is a common practice within many of these traditions. Divination is often used to prescribe ritualistic remedies for physical, emotional, mental, and spiritual ailments that are specific to the client. Unlike Abrahamic traditions that focus on a one-size-fits-all dogmatic approach to life, ATRs focus on taboos that are specific to each individual. For example, one person may be warned to avoid alcoholic beverages while another may be encouraged to eat plenty of meat. Focusing on individual recommendations allows these traditions to be customizable and change form over time. Though the same tradition may be practiced in different regions, specific rituals and remedies may vary. The transatlantic slave trade birthed several offshoots of Ifá in the Americas, each with their own rituals, songs, sacred dress, and food customs. Candomblé, Santería or Ocha, and Lukumi are all examples of different forms of Ifá across the diaspora. Though many of these traditions have similar practices, their differences separate them into distinct traditions.

Ifá was not the only ATR to be carried to the Americas. Vodou made its way to Haiti, Rastafarianism grew from Congolese and South Asian traditions, and Winti took root in Suriname. Within the United States, voodoo and hoodoo dominate the Black Southern tradition and continue to leave a lasting cultural and spiritual impact.

Haitian Vodou and Louisiana voodoo are two interconnected yet completely different traditions. Haitian Vodou draws many of its rituals, language, and food culture from West African *vodon,* an indigenous tradition practiced by the Aja, Ewe, and Fon peoples of Ghana, Benin, and Nigeria. The word *vodou* (also spelled voodoo, vodon) simply means "spirit." Similarly to Ifá, Haitian Vodou centers around the worship of *lwa,* spirits or gods that are deeply connected to the natural world. Louisiana voodoo, on the other hand, incorporates traditions from a range of different ethnic and cultural backgrounds, including Haitian Vodou, Congolese cosmology, Ifá, and Roman Catholicism. Both traditions have morphed and changed over time, adjusting to the sociopolitical context of the practitioners.

UNDERSTANDING THE WORLD THROUGH IFÁ

Unlike Christianity, Ifá describes a world that is much more nuanced and complicated. Concepts of good and evil are harder to disentangle from each other. Ifá teaches us that the true nature of the universe is multifaceted.

This multifacetedness extends to both nature and humans. Nature is neither good nor evil; it just is. In Southern California, wildfires often tear through communities, destroying homes and devastating families. While destruction is often in the wake of wildfires, so is rebirth. Wildfires clear necessary brush from the area and restart the ecological cycles that allow native plant life to thrive. To call a wildfire "evil" comes from a fallacy in your perspective. As humans, we tend to see the evil in things when they personally harm us. Ifá challenges us to decenter ourselves from our worldview and to instead recognize that we are one small piece in a system much larger than us. By shifting our perspective to that of other living beings around us, we see that good and evil don't truly exist.

Colonial mistranslations attempted to wipe out the wisdom of nuance that Ifá teaches us. One method is to "flatten" the inherent complexity of indigenous languages to fit a colonial worldview rooted in oversimplification. In Yoruba and in the Ifá tradition, Olódùmarè is the name or word for the supreme creator. It has been translated in English to mean "god." God in Christian cosmology is a relatively straightforward concept. God is the creator, god is masculine, god exists outside the universe because god is the creator of the universe. God exists outside humans, nature, plants, and animals. God is the ruler.

Prior to colonization, Yoruba was not a written language (see more on this in "A Note on Language" on page 21). When colonial translators attempted to document the linguistic complexities of the Yoruba language, they drew from their own worldview in an attempt to summarize a cosmology foreign from their own. In Yoruba, like many other languages, words are built by compounding several words together to create a new and unique meaning. When Olódùmarè is broken down into its individual parts, the Yoruba concept of the "creator" vastly contrasts the Euro-Christian perspective. Since Yoruba is traditionally a tonal oral language, different dialects are spoken across modern-day Benin and Nigeria. Sometimes these different dialects have slightly altered meanings for words, making Yoruba a deeply local dialect that intimately ties the speaker to their region of origin. Olódùmarè can also be spelled or pronounced as "Èlédùmàrè" or "Èdùmàrè." While Olódùmarè and Èlédùmàrè mean virtually the same thing, Èdùmàrè has a slightly different definition. In Yoruba, the prefixes *olo-* and *ele-* signify someone who possesses something, or someone who possesses the quality of that thing. For example, the word *olóko,* which combines the words *oló* (signifies possession) and *oko* (farm), means "farmer." In this example, *olóko* literally translates to "possessor or owner of the farm." In the word *eléwé,* the words *elé* (signifies possession) and *ewé* (leaf) come together to describe the color green, literally translating to "something that has the quality of a leaf."

When we break down *Olódùmarè* and *Èlédùmàrè* into their core parts, we're able to glean a deeper meaning beyond "creator." Combining the words *òdù* (pot or cauldron), *ma* (that does not), and *rè* (become exhausted of content or become finished), we get the phrase "pot or cauldron that never empties." The literal translation of *Olódùmarè* and *Èlédùmàrè* is "the owner pot or cauldron that never empties."[2] In Ifá cosmology, the universe is conceptualized as a calabash or bowl containing all possible realities.

Drawing from the translation of Olódùmarè or Èlédùmàrè, Ifá's concept of the universe is rooted in an ideal of abundance. Not only does the universe contain all possibilities, all positive and negative forces, and all life, but the universe is overflowing and infinite. When we break down *Èdùmàrè,* the word for the "creator" in a different regional Yoruba dialect, the meaning changes to "the pot that never empties." The subtle nuance in these two definitions is crucial. While *Olódùmarè* or *Èlédùmàrè* can either mean "the possessor of the pot that never empties" or "something that possesses a quality similar to a pot that never empties," *Èdùmàrè* specifically personifies the pot itself. Ifá does not necessarily view the creator as an entity separate from the universe, rather the creator is the universe itself. Ifá teaches us that the universe is infinite and overflowing, offering us an abundance of potential realities. Within this cosmology, both destructive and constructive forces exist within "Olódùmarè, Èlédùmàrè, Èdùmàrè, indicating that the creator is neither good nor bad. Olódùmarè just *is.*

The multifaceted nature of Olódùmarè can be seen within all aspects of the universe, because Olódùmarè is everything in the universe. As humans with a Western view of the world, we've been trained to believe that scientific study requires an objective view of the observable world. We're taught to believe that we can study "the universe" as if it exists somewhere outside of and separate from ourselves. To us, the universe is made up of stars, nebulas, galaxies, and planets zipping through space at alarming speeds. Ifá, similarly to many other indigenous cosmologies around the world, views humans as an integral part of the universe. We are not able to study the universe objectively because we are the universe itself. In Ifá the orisas represent different aspects of nature or different natural phenomena. Like Olódùmarè, the orisas are multifaceted, complicated forces that don't fall neatly into the categories of good and evil.

Perhaps the best-known and most misrepresented orisa, Esu most clearly represents both the multifaceted and unpredictable nature of the orisas. Known by many names, including Elégbà, Elegua, Legba, and the Crossroads Man, Esu is the orisa of possibility. He's personified as both a childish young boy and a mysterious old man. During masquerade performances, performers representing Esu sometimes wear women's clothing while parading around large phalluses, embodying the playful and mischievous nature of the orisa. Esu is known generally as the trickster, leading to mixed messaging about his true nature.

Unlike Christianity, there are no orisas that go against Olódùmarè. Since Olódùmarè is the embodiment of everything in the universe, the orisas can be understood to be just one of Olódùmarè's many aspects. Esu's role in Yoruba cosmology is to communicate with both the light and dark forces within the universe. Esu's ability to communicate with all the forces in the universe is represented by his role as guardian of the crossroads, the one we consult when we need to make a decision. Esu can open and close all paths that lead to all possibilities in the universe. By communicating with all forces, Esu can appease both the negative and positive forces in the universe, helping to guide us down our desired path.

Esu's misrepresentation began when Samuel Ajayi Crowther, a formerly enslaved Yoruba man who was later baptized and became a leading missionary, mistranslated Esu during his attempt to assign an existing Yoruba deity to Satan in the Christian Bible.[3] His misassignment began the centuries-long misrepresentation of Esu as dark and evil. Songs about selling your soul to the devil at the crossroads, like the popular hoodoo song by Robert Johnson, can be traced back to Crowther.

In Yoruba, Esu is more commonly known as Elégbà. Through the Hispanicization of the Yoruba language because of the transatlantic slave trade, Elégbà became Elegua among Spanish-speaking Lukumi and Santería practitioners. When we break down *Elégbà* into discrete parts, we're left with *ele*, meaning "the one who possesses (the quality of)," and *gba*, meaning "receive," "collect," or "(come to the) rescue (of)." Elégbà is the one who receives and rescues.[4] When Ifá practitioners offer ebo, or sacrifice, Esu is the one that carries their prayers and sacrifices to the corresponding orisas or other forces in the universe. Ebo comes in many forms, and often includes *obi*, or kola nuts. Esu takes sacrifices and uses them as bargaining chips on the behalf of the person giving ebo. Ifá is built on a system of reciprocity. You cannot ask for something without giving something in return. Esu represents this system of reciprocity and balance.

CONNECTING BLACK TRADITIONS THROUGH THE DIASPORA

Although I've been focusing on the linguistic aspects of Ifá, this book is not a linguistic mapping of West African traditions. My goal in breaking down the core aspects of blessing in Ifá, Olódùmarè, and Esu is to illustrate the ways concepts in Ifá can be and are currently used as frameworks that guide Black life across the diaspora. So many aspects of Ifá are rooted in a community-centered approach. Hierarchies exist within the tradition, but many of the teachings are rooted in a deep understanding of community that extends to the ancestral realm and to nature. Ifá teaches us that we are not individuals and that we cannot achieve anything alone; rather we are one aspect of a multifaceted web that relies on itself to survive. Ifá teaches us the importance of interdependence.

In *Wayward Lives, Beautiful Experiments,* Saidiya Hartman explores the ways Black queer life in urban city centers at the turn of the twentieth century was rooted in a form of Black anarchy driven by improvisation and a desire to do more than simply survive. She explores the ways Black women rewrote the rules of society within the "Black ghetto," attracting the attention of sociologists and reporters who were both horrified and fascinated by the Black urban experience. The narratives and images taken from this period create a "poverty porn" phenomenon surrounding Black life. What Saidiya explores is the beauty, ingenuity, anarchism, and life that blossoms outside of the sociologists' and reporters' accounts. She explores "the beauty of black ordinary, the beauty that resides in and animates the determination to live free, the beauty that propels the experiments in living otherwise."[5] Through her study of Black women and Black queer people, Saidiya explains that "beauty is not a luxury; rather it is a way of creating possibility in the space of enclosure, a radical art of subsistence, an embrace of our terribleness, a transfiguration of the given. It is a will to adorn, a proclivity for the baroque, and the love of *too much*."

What does it mean to have a love of *too much* in a universe that is built on a concept of abundance? The inherent beauty in Black life that Saidiya describes comes from a complex mix of pain, art, and determination. When I first read Saidiya's words, I was reminded of the way the concept of Olódùmarè and Esu fully encompass this interplay between the grime and muck and the divine and beautiful, and how this interplay is the foundation of the Black experience.

In *Of Water and the Spirit: Ritual, Magic, and Initiation in the Life of an African Shaman*, Malidoma Patrice Somé examines the interplay between the ugliness and beauty of life. While cleanliness is linked to godliness within Western religion and culture, the Dagara people hold the opposite belief to be true. Before life can produce beauty and sweetness, it must first produce ugliness and rot. Malidoma's grandfather explained to him at an early age that sweet floral fragrances are born from horrible ones. He explains that before a flower can produce a sweet smell, it must first rot.[6] Within Dagara culture, beauty in the aesthetic sense is deprioritized. Throughout the book, Malidoma describes the appearance of Dagara spiritual leaders as disheveled and unkempt, a sign that their priorities are focused on their deep spiritual connection with the world around them rather than with aesthetic beauty. This theme can be seen in Ifá as well, as exemplified by Yoruba shrines. Traditional Yoruba shrines are often covered in alcohol, kola nuts, food, palm oil, and blood. Though they may be in beautiful places, the shrines themselves are not traditionally aesthetically pleasing. Shrines within the Ifá tradition are centers of power for the orisa. They represent a sacred meeting point where Ifá practitioners and the orisas can communicate.

As I read these passages from *Of Water and the Spirit*, I thought of all the beauty that has grown out of struggle, hardship, and brutality. I thought of Black queer chosen families formed in the wake of abandonment. I thought of BIPOC urban farms and community gardens where the requirement for multigenerational knowledge-sharing is quite literally getting your hands dirty. Malidoma's words reminded me of the beauty that lies within the ordinary.

Both Saidiya Hartman and William C. Anderson explore the beauty and complexity that lies within ordinary Black life. In *The Nation on No Map: Black Anarchism and Abolition,* Anderson discusses the fantasies many Black Americans tell themselves about who their ancestors were. Many of these fantasies center around royal lineage and seek to highlight examples of Black nation-building that most resembles the kings and queens of Europe. Anderson argues that these fantasies create a harmful mythos that disregards the ordinary Black lives the majority of our ancestors lived. He states that "Black Americans must confront the truths about who we actually are *now* rather than fabricating counterproductive tales about who we were *then*."[7] Leaning into Anderson's argument, I want to highlight the realities of ordinary Black life, both then and now. My goal is to uplift the "cheap socialism," as Hartman calls it, that colors so much of Black life, both past and present. Through the lens of Black spirituality, I want to showcase the beauty that Black people have created and honor the lives of the ordinary people that made it possible.

IFÁ AS A FRAMEWORK

This book will illustrate the ways culture has traveled and transformed across the African diaspora using my understanding of Ifá as a framework. Drawing from my ilé's perspective and teachings of Ifá, I want to explore the ways the five blessings in Ifá (longevity, wealth, partnership, children, and victory) show up in Black life across the diaspora. I hope to illustrate the unique ways Black people have held on to our culture and traditions and transformed them to fit the demands of Black life when faced with white supremacy and climate change. As someone born in the United States to Black American parents, much of my analysis and understanding will inherently be from a Black American perspective. Where I fall short, I hope to draw from prominent writers and spiritual leaders that are embedded within aspects of the diaspora that I am less familiar with. I will draw from my experience in both biology and anthropology to map African traditional views onto Black modern struggles such as the fight for food sovereignty and the creation of Black queer spaces.

This is not a religious text or an overview of Ifá as a tradition. My goal is not to encourage readers to practice Ifá or any other Afro-Indigenous spiritual tradition. Cultural appropriation and spiritual co-opting are two phenomena I actively fight against. Ifá is first and foremost a Black African spiritual tradition. Many babalawos and iyanifas feel that this tradition belongs only to Black African people and their descendants. What I hope readers take away from this book is not dogma, but a deeper understanding of the beauty and complexity of Black life and culture. I want readers to understand that even though most Black people do not practice ATRs, the frameworks within them continue to guide the ways Black people build community, structure our families, and protect the natural world around us.

It's important to note that Ifá, like many indigenous spiritual traditions, is sacred and much of the teachings are kept hidden from the public. I have not undergone full initiation into the tradition, so much of Ifá's deeper teachings remain unknown to me. None of the information I plan to share in this book will divulge any closely kept spiritual traditions. I ask that curious readers exercise respect and restraint when researching further into any indigenous spiritual tradition. The keepers of Ifá are the iyanifas and babalawos who undergo years of rigorous study to commit odus to memory and dedicate their lives to upholding this tradition. This is not something you can learn overnight. For anyone interested in understanding Ifá on a deeper level, it's important to understand the years of dedication required to enter this tradition. I ask that all readers respect this and respect the boundaries iyanifas and babalawos set about who does and does not have access to this practice.

READING THIS BOOK

This book will focus on all the Black beauty and triumph that was born out of and despite brutality, white supremacy, and colonial forces. I plan to showcase the inventive and imaginative ways Black people across the diaspora have carved out places we can call home and turned lemons into lemonade. As a collective, we've managed to usher in the five blessings of Ifá into our lives despite all odds. This book is a love letter and a guide. I hope to illustrate what's possible by reminding us of what we've already accomplished.

In the first chapter, I'll discuss the blessing of Ire Àìkú, the blessing of longevity. I'll compare ancestral herbalism and urban farming, highlighting the ways both practices are rooted in the concept of legacy. Referencing both Leah Penniman's and Michele E. Lee's work, I'll discuss the ways our ancestral traditions have stood the test of time while our new and inventive forms of sustainability and food sovereignty in the modern world provide us with a path forward for future generations. I'll explore the concept of food sovereignty across the diaspora, diving into a range of topics from the Black vegan movement in the United States, *ital* food within the Rastafari religion in Jamaica, and innovative farming techniques across the African continent.

In the second chapter, I'll discuss the blessing of Ire Àjé, the blessing of wealth. This chapter will focus on the wealth and richness of the communities we've created. I'll explore Black queer and trans communities, Candomblé and Capoeira in Brazil, and the Black church. Drawing from Saidiya Hartman's and William C. Anderson's work, I'll explore the power of community and the importance of social capital as a tool for Black survival. Food, dance, and music serve as threads that connect seemingly disparate African diasporic cultures together into one. The richness and depth of these cultural traditions is the truest form of wealth and most exemplifies the blessing of Ire Àjé.

In the third chapter, I'll discuss the blessing of Ire Ọkọ/Aya, the blessing of husband/wife. This chapter will take a nontraditional view of marriage and partnership, focusing on a variety of relationship structures, including the relationship between Black parents and children, Black queer relationships, and ancestral relationships that span generations. By breaking down the multifaceted linguistic meanings of both ọkọ and aya, I'll argue that queer and alternative relationship structures have a long and rich history in West Africa. Using research from Oyèrónkẹ́ Oyěwùmí, I'll compare indigenous relationship structures to more modern queer relationships.

In the fourth chapter, I'll discuss the blessing of Ire Ọmọ, the blessing of children. Here, I'll explore both alternative birthing practices and child-rearing techniques. Drawing from my own experience as a doula in training and from the wisdom of doulas I've had the opportunity to work with, I'll dive into the history of Black doulas and midwives and discuss how their resurgence is a means to combat the high Black maternal mortality rate in the United States. I'll discuss the rise of gentle parenting among a new generation of Black parents seeking to heal their inner child and break the cycle of generational trauma. I'll explore the role of Black parents in maintaining traditions and culture and discuss the ways alternative family structures can expand our capacity to know ourselves and each other.

In the fifth chapter, I'll discuss the blessing of Ire Ìṣẹ́gun, victory over negative forces. I'll focus on Black autonomy in all its forms, both past and present. This chapter will first take a historical look at revolutionary "slave revolts," including the Haitian Revolution and the Stono Rebellion. From there, I'll connect the Black beauty movement to the Black power movement at large, emphasizing the importance of mutual aid in Black autonomous resistance in the United States. I'll conclude this chapter by exploring the Black witch movement as a modern-day resistance against Christian hegemony, particularly for Black women and queer and trans people.

A NOTE ON LANGUAGE

Ifá is an indigenous spiritual tradition from the Yoruba people in modern-day Nigeria, Benin, and the surrounding regions. Both from the oral nature of the Yoruba language and the colonial forces on language that resulted from the transatlantic slave trade, many of the Yoruba spellings have become Hispanicized and Anglicized. For example, most Yoruba spellings use tonal marks to denote complex sounds, while Spanish and English tend to rely on consonant pairs. This is most evident with Yoruba words that have a "sh" sound. The common Yoruba spelling is *Ọṣun,* while the Anglicized spelling is *Oshun.* Another example is the difference in the Yoruba spelling for *orisa* compared to the Anglicized spelling *orisha.* Both spellings are accurate, and one is not more correct than the other. In Spanish dialects, the "sh" sound is often replaced by *ch.* Some examples include the Yoruba spelling of *Ṣàngó* and orisa compared to the Lukumi spelling of *Chango* and *oricha.*

A different phenomenon arises when Yoruba words are spoken within Spanish or Portuguese dialects. Since Yoruba was initially an oral language with no written tradition, the language was carried phonetically around the world. As dialects and languages changed among enslaved Africans, so did the pronunciations of Yoruba words. The Yoruba *Elégbà* became the Hispanicized *Elegua.* The Hispanicization of Yoruba words extends beyond the names for the orisas. In Portuguese, the "sh" sound is spelled with *x,* so the Yoruba *Ọṣun* becomes the Portuguese *Oxum.*

A comparison of Yoruba orisas with New World linguistic differences and Vodou equivalents. Source: *The Handbook of Yoruba Religious Concepts*[8]

YORUBA IFÁ ORIṢA	SANTERÍA AND LUKUMI ORISA	CANDOMBLÉ ORIXA	VODOU LWA OR LOA
Eṣu	Elegua	Exu	Legba
Ọbàtálá	Obatala	Oxalá	Batala, Blanc Dani
Yemọja	Yemayá	Iemanjá	Agwe, La Baili-anne, Yemalla
Ọṣun	Ochun	Oxum	Erzuli
Ògún	Ogún	Ogum	Ogu, Gu, Oguoun
Oshoosi	Ochossi	Oxossi	Age

YORUBA IFÁ ORIṢA	SANTERÍA AND LUKUMI ORISA	CANDOMBLÉ ORIXA	VODOU LWA OR LOA
Osain	Osain	Ossaim	Erinle
Ṣàngó	Chango	Xango	Xevioso
Ọya	Ọya	Ọya, Iansa	Aieda-Lenso, Olla
Bablu-aye	Babalu-Aye	Omolu, Babaluiye	Sakpata
Olokun	Olokun	Olokun	Agwe, Mami Wata

Throughout this book, I use the Yoruba spelling as a form of linguistic mapping. I derive sociocultural analyses by breaking down Yoruba concepts into foundational worlds. I then reconstruct the original word based on its foundational definitions and use those concepts to construct a worldview based in Yoruba dialect. Although this book is not a purely linguistic analysis, understanding the linguistic components of African diasporic cultures is crucial to understanding Black and African spiritual and political movements. When relevant, I will draw attention to alternative spellings for key concepts so as not to confuse readers who may have knowledge of other ATRs.

1

THE BLESSING OF ÀÌKÚ

If some people forget their past as a way to survive,
other people remember it for the same reason.
—MALIDOMA PATRICE SOMÉ, *OF WATER AND THE SPIRIT*

When I was in eleventh grade, I was assigned a family tree project for school. I'd done several of these projects over the years, and I dreaded the assignment every time. Family history projects always filled me with a mix of anxiety, shame, and frustration. Growing up in a predominantly white neighborhood in Orange County, California, I was usually one of the few Black kids in my classes. Both my maternal and paternal grandparents were originally from the South and had moved to Los Angeles in the 1950s during the Second Great Migration. Beginning in 1910 and ending in the 1970s, Black people left the South to flee racist violence and in search of better economic opportunities in two major waves known collectively as the Great Migration. My mother's parents moved to South Los Angeles on the border between the Compton and Gardena neighborhoods while my father's parents settled in Inglewood. As children, both my parents took frequent trips to the South, visiting family in Alabama, Texas, and Florida. As a child, my only connection to the South was through stories my parents and grandparents told, leaving me feeling unmoored and disconnected from my family's history.

Most of the nonwhite kids I grew up with were first- or second-generation immigrants whose parents or grandparents had immigrated to the United States. I was too young to fully understand the ways US imperialism and economic warfare pushed many of my peers' families to leave their countries of origin in search of better opportunities. When they spoke about their connection to land, culture, and community abroad, I felt ashamed about my lack of clarity about my family's history. Though most of the white kids in class didn't have direct ties to family outside of the United States, many of them had meticulous records of their relatives. One classmate boasted about going to France and finding old marriage certificates from his relatives dating back to the 1300s.

All of my family records were passed down orally or written down in the pages of my grandmother Louise's Bible and phone book. My mom, aunt, and grandmother would recount stories of relatives who I never met or was too young to remember, laughing about memories from their childhoods spent in Alabama. Both my maternal grandmother, Louise, one of nine children, and my grandfather, Johnny, grew up around the corner from each other in Union Springs, Alabama. Louise's mother, Sallie Mae, started the first Black kindergarten in Union Springs and taught my grandfather Johnny in one of her classes. Their stories about Union Springs were filled with life, colored by all the relatives and friends that lived nearby.

My paternal grandparents rarely spoke about their childhoods. When my paternal grandfather, Lawrence, was about six years old, both his parents tragically passed away. He and his four siblings moved in with their aunt and uncle, who had several children of their own. My grandfather grew up in South Carolina as a descendant of the Gullah Geechee people, a sub-ethnic group of African Americans with a unique linguistic and culinary culture that developed from enslaved Africans who formed communities along the Carolina coast and the neighboring Sea Islands. My paternal grandmother, Sandra, was adopted as a young child and didn't reconnect with many of her relatives until later in life. Although she grew up in Texas, her biological family was originally from Louisiana. My dad remembers meeting his grandfather, Louis Tassin, and his great-grandmother, Adine Bush. Both Louis and Adine predominantly spoke Creole, making it difficult to cross the language barrier and build a deeper connection. Both of my paternal grandparents' childhoods left them separated from parts of their family history. From the stories told to me by my parents and grandparents, I pieced together a tapestry of history that connected me to Alabama, Louisiana, and the Sea Islands.

When I was in high school, Ancestry.com had recently launched their DNA testing service, claiming to link people to specific regions around the world based on their DNA test results. My dad became obsessed with the quest to understand his ancestry, spending hours sifting through records on Ancestry.com, obsessively watching Henry Louis Gates Jr.'s show *Finding Your Roots* on PBS, and eventually buying the Ancestry.com DNA test kit for himself. I had mixed feelings about my father's interest in his ancestry. I grew up with stories about my Gullah Geechee great-grandparents from my grandfather Lawrence and my Creole great-grandfather from my grandmother Sandra. Since both my grandparents were disconnected from their biological parents when they were young, I was left with more questions about my dad's side of the family. I was hopeful that an Ancestry DNA test might provide my family with a clearer picture of our heritage. On the other hand, I was anxious about handing over my DNA to a corporation, especially since it was unknown how these companies might use the data they collect.

I was also anxious about what information I would find about my non-Black ancestors. As a descendant from enslaved Africans, I knew I had some non-Black ancestry. Part of the violence of colonialism and enslavement was the sexual assault of Black women. It's a part of my history that filled me with uneasiness and rage. My grandmother and father prided themselves on their Louisiana roots and the "French" heritage that they claimed gave us our straight noses. "You have a beautiful nose," my grandmother always said. "Other Black girls are jealous of noses like yours." Growing up, I felt self-conscious about my nose, feeling that it didn't quite fit the features of my face. But hearing my grandmother connect my nose to France filled me with a complicated mix of emotions. France was a country with an overabundance of history and culture that was widely accessible to me. As a kid, I studied French in school and had a Parisian-themed bedroom. It felt a twinge of pride in being distantly connected to a culture I romanticized in my childhood fantasies. I understood the desire to be in closer proximity to whiteness from a very young age, even if I didn't have the language to articulate that desire. I saw it from my grandmother Louise, who claimed that her long hair was attributed to her Indigenous American ancestry, a common belief held by many African Americans. I saw it from my mother, who rolled her eyes and mocked my father every time he mentioned his Gullah Geechee heritage. I saw it from my cousins, who would compare their skin tone to mine, making fun of me for being darker or claiming I would be prettier if I was light like them. These early messages from my childhood gave me mixed signals about how to feel about my ancestry.

Despite the mixed signals my family sent about my heritage, they were always proud to be Black. I knew I was Black through and through, and when I was with my family, I felt proud of my heritage. Even though my family claimed to trace their roots to other racial and ethnic groups, they never viewed themselves as anything other than Black, specifically African American. My parents and grandparents worked hard to instill a sense of pride in my identity. Spending time with my family was a balm for the hurt and insecurities I developed from the racist bullying I endured at school. At school I was ugly. My hair was too short and my skin was too dark. Students would whisper slurs as I walked down the halls to see if I would react. When I was in seventh grade, a group of students poured water on my newly pressed hair while I waited after school for my mom to pick me up. Their bullying ate away at me, planting the seeds for early childhood depression and insecurities that filled me with self-doubt.

At home, it was a different story. My parents and grandparents constantly showered me in praise for my academic achievements. My mother, grandmother, and great-grandmother all worked in K-12 education. My mom and grandmother always instilled in me the importance of doing well in school. "That girl is smart as a whip," my grandmother Louise would often affectionately say. I grew up with home-cooked meals, gospel music, and holidays spent in my grandmother's house with all my cousins, aunts, and uncles. I have fond memories of watching my mom and grandmother cook Thanksgiving dinner. They prepared an assortment of dishes, including candied yams, stuffing, and German chocolate cake.

My summer breaks were spent at my aunt's house, running around with my cousins. My childhood was spent running through the waves at Huntington Beach, searching for Dippin' Dots at Knott's Berry Farm, and watching TV in my grandmother's garage. Though I had fun spending time with my friends and my cousins, I felt isolated in Orange County. I felt the most at home in Los Angeles in my grandmother's garden. My grandmother and I would spend hours making crafts with pipe cleaners, hot glue, and pompoms. The overwhelming love I received from her filled me with joy. I was proud to be Black because I wanted to be more like her.

My dad was overjoyed when I asked for his help on my family tree assignment. He pulled up records from Ancestry.com, excited to show me how much he'd been able to compile over the years, what he'd pieced together from the fragmented history of our family. He collected census records, marriage certificates, and obituaries. He pored over slave records indicating just the age, sex, and race (either negro or mulatto) of the enslaved person, speculating whether the "F, 29, negro" was an ancestor of ours. I was impressed by how far he'd been able to come on his quest for understanding. I was fascinated by the number of people in my family tree and the complicated history many of my ancestors had in terms of their relationship to the United States. One ancestor fought in the Civil War while another married a Confederate soldier. Some ancestors were able to buy their freedom and the freedom of their loved ones, while others remained enslaved and displaced across the American South. Parsing the records reinforced my father's pride in his parents' Southern roots. When I asked my father where our family was from, he'd say, "Your people are from the South," proudly emphasizing the rich and complex culture that tied my family together.

Until I started writing this book, I had never gone to Union Springs, where my maternal grandmother and grandfather were raised. So when my mother asked me and my brother if we wanted to go on a family trip to Alabama in March 2024, I seized the opportunity. My parents, brother, a few aunts and uncles, and I spent a week visiting my grandmother Louise's and grandfather Johnny's families in Alabama and Georgia. During our trip, we attended a distant cousin's wedding, visited my great-aunt Lucille, and drove around my grandparent's childhood neighborhood. On our last day in Alabama we attended a church service at the church my grandparents and their siblings attended in their youth. After the service we drove up the street to my great-uncle Buddy's house. Uncle Buddy was my grandmother's oldest brother. When he was in better health, he had a small farm on his property where he grew a few staple crops and raised chickens; he mailed peanuts to his younger sister, my grandmother Louise. News of our visit led to an impromptu family reunion. Some of my relatives lived next door to Uncle Buddy in Sallie Mae's old house or in one of the adjacent houses. Others drove from Birmingham and Atlanta to greet us. The tiny house was packed with cousins, aunts, and uncles laughing, chatting, and cooking. I sat on the sofa with my second cousin Amber as she flipped through photo albums and pointed out different relatives to help my brother and me understand how we were all related. Visiting my family's neighborhood in Alabama allowed me to locate my family's history in a physical place. For the first time, it felt like my history was rooted in a tangible place, somewhere I could call my ancestral home. I finally had somewhere I could return to.

There's a long history of shame associated with African American heritage and culture as a result of enslavement and systematic racism and discrimination. For many Black families, our knowledge of our ancestors is fragmented, pieced together from stories and family myths. The violent process of enslavement, the specific geography of the South, and the unique form white supremacy took within the United States created a hostile environment for African cultures to take root and thrive. Unlike the Caribbean and Latin America, a relatively small percentage of enslaved Africans were transported to the United States. These numbers and the particular US system of slavery and Jim Crow segregation following slavery both created a particularly oppressive environment that sought to stamp out all aspects of African American heritage and culture. Though Black Americans have retained much of their West African roots and have gone on to create a thriving and vibrant culture that is globally recognized and appreciated today, dominant narratives that reinforce shame in one's background continue to persist.

Keeping my grandparents' memory alive is an important aspect of archiving my family's history. So many Black families have fragmented family stories, with bits and pieces of history scattered or lost to time. Contextualizing my grandparents' and great-grandparents' lives with the history of African American people helps me heal generations of disconnection.

THE IMPORTANCE OF OUR ANCESTORS

Ancestors are at the heart of ATRs and African diasporic religions (ADRs). Before any communication with the orisa or lwa can be made, you first have to connect with ancestors. *Egún or egúngún* (*eégún* for short) is the Yoruba word for ancestor. When we break the word down further, *gún* means "to arrive," "to align," or "to pound, pierce, or stab," depending on the context. In this context, *gún* refers more to the meanings of "to arrive" and "to align." Putting it all together, *egún* means "the ones who arrive (to align)."[1] This speaks to the role ancestors play in the traditional practice of Ifá. Ancestors are often called upon to provide guidance within the lives of the practitioners. They serve as a powerful first connector between the visible and invisible forces.

In *African Cosmology of the Bântu-Kôngo: Tying the Spiritual Knot,* Fu-Kiau describes the Kongo cosmogram, the Bantu-Kongo map of the flow of the universe. Within Kongo cosmology, the universe and everything in it is composed of energy that's "living" in some form or another. The world can be understood as two planes of existence: the physical world and the spiritual world. Both planes are connected through the cycle of birth and death and are separated by the *kalunga.*

There are four main life stages in Kongo cosmology, each with a corresponding color: *musoni, kala, tukula,* and *luvemba.* Musoni, represented by the color yellow, is the time spent in the spirit world or ancestral world. This realm is described as a forest: dark, mysterious, full of knowledge, but also disorienting and easy to get lost or misguided in. The time spent in this zone is immeasurable because time operates differently in this plane of existence. Once enough knowledge has been acquired in the spirit-ancestral realm, the next stage is rebirth, or kala, represented by the color black. Blackness represents the emergence of life. Tukula, represented by the color red, is marked by growth and maturity as well as mastery of one's skills and talents in young adulthood. This is the stage when you truly step into yourself and your purpose. This is also the stage of leadership and using your skills to better your community and the world around you. How you behave during the tukula stage determines how you will experience the ancestral realm and whether or not you will return. Those who are lost spiritually will turn into lost spirits upon death. *N'kuyu* are "bad ancestors" or lost spirits who aimlessly wander the ancestral realm. Luvemba, represented by the color white, is death. Leading up to this phase, leaders in the community pass on their knowledge to younger generations, often through initiations.[2] White represents death and the spiritual realm in many West African traditions. The white cloth used for ancestor altars alludes to this symbolism.

Constructing an ancestor altar is a crucial part of any ATR or ADR. Many cultures around the world venerate ancestors in similar ways, usually leaving offerings of some kind for the dead. In ATRs and ADRs, ancestor altars are usually composed of three main components. The first is laying a white cloth on some sort of designated surface. It can be your dresser, a table, or even the floor.

The second component of an ancestor altar is a glass of water. In many West African cultures, water acts as a portal and conduit for communicating with the dead.[3] Across cultures, water is deeply connected to spirituality because of its life-giving properties. Water or *omi* is reflective, representing the duality of oneself and nature. Water is said to hold memory, making it the perfect tool to help connect to the memories of our ancestors. Water is also cooling, helping us keep a cool head and release pent-up anger and rage when we come to our ancestor altar. Water is also a portal, allowing us to connect with realms beyond our own. Freshwater specifically is associated with Ọṣun, the orisa of sweet waters, the mother of fishes, and the patron of healers. Water is typically changed out every few days to keep it fresh and free of dust and debris. Some people view water as an offering to ancestors, while others view it strictly as a tool for communication.

The third component of an ancestor altar is a white candle. Candles are commonly used in spiritual practices as a way to concentrate energy or to help get things moving energetically. Fire, an element associated with Ṣàngó, brings vitality to your ancestor altar. It helps reignite the connection between the living and the dead, working with water to serve as a conduit for communication.

When I began my practice of Ifá, I was eager to tap into the "more authentic" spiritual traditions from West Africa. Spiritual and cultural exports from West Africa felt more authentic to me because they were presumably less influenced by colonial forces than African American traditions. To me, West African practices had a purity that I didn't associate with Black American traditions. I diminished the traditions of my most recent Black American ancestors, the hoodoo and voodoo that I had been researching for years, because they felt watered down compared to traditions like Ifá and Lukumi. Despite my study of Black culture, I fell into the trap of discounting Black American traditions the same way my parents and grandparents had. Those biases continued to live on within my psyche, pushing me away from Black American traditions in search of something that felt "more grounded" and somehow more ancestral.

Thus, I was shocked when my first assignment from my iyanifa was to construct a family tree. Long out of K-12 schooling, I thought I'd finally escaped the embarrassment and dread that came with reconstructing my family lineage. My iyanifa instructed me to write down a list of as many names as I could from both my mother and father's lineage. She also instructed me to collect as many old photographs of deceased relatives as I could and to include them on my ancestor altar. Reluctantly, I spent a few weeks digging through records my father shared with me on Ancestry.com, looking for names of relatives. Since high school, I hadn't taken the time to look through my family tree in any detail.

When I first constructed my ancestor altar, I was more concerned with the aesthetics of the altar than its functionality. Ancestor altars do not need to be elaborately decorated and shouldn't be expensive to create. Caught up in the image of spirituality, I covered my dresser in a white tapestry with a mandala print in the center, bought several big white candles, and filled the space with crystals and trinkets that I valued more for their beauty than their spiritual properties. My altar was clogged up with items that had no personal connection to me or my ancestors. It was also difficult to clean and take care of because all the extra crystals and candles accumulated dust. As time went on, the difficulty of maintaining such an elaborate altar led me to come to my altar less and less. I rarely changed the water or left offerings. What was supposed to be a space for cultivating a deeper connection with my ancestry became a place of clutter and dread.

I unintentionally filled my altar space with feelings of dread because internally that was how I felt going into the assignment; my own complicated feelings about my relationship to my ancestors spilled out onto the physical space. I focused on the material aspect of the altar to shield myself from having to delve deeper into the interpersonal and spiritual aspects of my practice. At this point in my journey, I focused on reaching a particular destination rather than immersing myself in practice. I treated each new lesson as a means to an end. I applied the same academic mindset that allowed me to excel in higher education to my spiritual practices. I thought that if I could fly through each assignment, I'd be on my way to priestesshood in no time. I've since learned that indigenous spirituality is about slowing down. These practices take a lifetime to learn, so there's no reason to rush the process.

My biggest lesson in slowing down came with the passing of my grandfather Johnny and grandmother Louise in 2018 and 2019. I dealt with the grief in dramatically different ways. Unlike my grandfather's death, I was mentally prepared for my grandmother's. My grandmother had been suffering from Alzheimer's and dementia for ten years, giving me plenty of time to come to terms with her illness. My grandfather passed away rather suddenly after he fell and hit his head right before New Year's Eve, leading to a rapid health decline. When his health took a turn for the worse, my grandfather moved into my parents' home to live out his final days. I heard of his passing while I was away at college. My parents decided that it was best for me to focus on school and decided that I didn't need to come home for the funeral. It felt like I didn't have an opportunity to properly process his passing.

My grandfather was the first relative I knew, and one of the first people I was close to, to pass away. A few weeks after the funeral, I broke out in hives all over my body. My skin became red and inflamed and my lips swelled, landing me in and out of the hospital for two weeks. I was put on steroid medications to help with the inflammation, but they only made it worse. Doctors asked me if I had any allergies or if there was any sudden stress that could have triggered an autoimmune response. The only thing that came to mind was the death of my grandfather. Until then, I had felt numb and detached from his passing. Even if I didn't have conscious access to those emotions, the stress was manifesting in my body. Even though the initial outbreak subsided, I still sporadically develop hives and swollen lips whenever I am stressed.

The toll my grandfather's death took on my body led me to herbalism and spirituality in search of natural remedies and grounding practices to help regulate my stress and address the symptoms of my flare-ups. I'd always been interested in natural remedies, but I began to pay closer attention to my relationship with my body. Incorporating my knowledge of plant-based eating and natural hair care, I embarked on my herbalism and spirituality journey.

ANCESTRAL RELATING

In Ifá specifically and African spiritual systems generally, being an ancestor is a status that's earned. To be an ancestor in death, you have to be actively working toward the betterment of yourself and your community during your lifetime. Becoming an ancestor means you are remembered and honored after your death, and that when invoked, your spirit brings warmth, healing, and energy to your community. Invoking someone's spirit sounds complicated, but it simply means to call upon the memory and legacy of that person and to remember their contributions to their family and community. Ancestors are more than your direct relatives. They also refer to your spiritual family and community.

Understanding where you came from is crucial to understand where you are going. Ifá is all about the path or destiny that one is meant to follow in their lifetime. Many forces have conspired to bring each of us to where we are today. One's ancestors are the most obvious force, since they are the people whose DNA makes up your body. In a way, the genetic transfer of DNA is a form of reincarnation. In Ifá, rebirth is a central concept and is said to happen within family lines. Your ancestors continue to live on within you, and their spirit continues to influence your life. When we think of generational trauma, that can be said to be a form of our ancestors' pain continuing to impact our lives. I bring up generational trauma because not all of our ancestors lived fulfilling and happy lives, and not all of them were people who contributed to their communities and families in a constructive way. As the descendants of enslaved Africans, many Black diasporans have complicated ancestry that includes overseers and enslavers. We can acknowledge this painful history and still honor and uplift the ancestors that left an overall positive mark on our families.

People new to these traditions start off by leaving offerings for their ancestors as a way to build a deeper connection with them. Leaving offerings for ancestors is relatively simple. Typically, offerings of food are left on ancestor altars, but other offerings like coffee and tobacco are popular as well. Whenever I cook a meal I know my relatives loved, I leave a little plate for them at the altar.

In Ifá, Vodou, Candomblé, and Lukumi, interacting with the orisa or lwa is not a simple task. It requires deep study that takes a lifetime to truly master how to interact with the divine forces of nature. The average person cannot give offerings to, or "feed," the orisa or lwa during ceremony; only someone who is dedicated to undergoing the initiation process can engage with this process.

When an apprentice—ọmọ awo, which literally translates to "child of mystery"—begins to work with the orisa, the first orisa many work with is Ifá, also known as Ọ̀rúnmìlà. In Isese, ọmọ awo receive Ifá during a sacred ceremony. This process is referred to as receiving your "Hand of Ifá" and requires the work of a babalawo or iyanifa. After receiving their Hand of Ifá, ọmọ awos become aborisas, devotees of Ifá. There are many sacred components to this ceremony, and some of those components differ by tradition. Most commonly, aborisas receive their *ilẹkẹs* (also spelled *elekes*), which are sacred beads representing specific orisa. The word *ilẹkẹs* means "bead" in

Yoruba. These beads are strung by sacred beaders and are consecrated by babalawos or iyanifas specifically for the aborisa. During this ceremony, the orisa that "owns your head" is also revealed.

The goal of receiving your Hand of Ifá is to work to ensure Ire Àìkú, the blessing of longevity. Receiving one's Hand of Ifá bestows the blessings of Ọ̀rúnmìlà. When done in person, an aborisa receives a special *ide*, or bracelet, known as an *idefá*, which identifies them as a child of Ọ̀rúnmìlà. As a child of Ọ̀rúnmìlà, *iku*, or death, does not have the ability to take them without Ọ̀rúnmìlà's permission.[4] The Hand of Ifá ceremony is a crucial first step in averting death and helping to ensure a long life for the initiate.

Another aspect of the ceremony is learning which orisa is the owner of the ọmọ awo's head. Depending on which orisa owns one's head, the ọmọ awo will be given a list of taboos that are important for them to follow for their health and safety. Unlike many dogmatic traditions, Ifá tends to take a prescriptive approach to spirituality. Through divination, one's taboos are revealed. Everyone has a different list that can include warnings against eating certain foods, drinking certain liquors, wearing certain colors, or participating in certain activities. Breaking a taboo could result in a number of *osogbo*, negative forces, including misfortune, illness, and death. By adhering to the advice given during divination, the ọmọ awo can work to avoid osogbo and ensure as much *ire* as possible manifests in their life.

After receiving one's Ifá, the aborisa begins the process of learning to "make ose," the ritual feeding of one's Ifá shrine. Each orisa shrine is fed differently on different days corresponding to the Yoruba calendar, which consists of four-day weeks and seven-week months. On Ifá's day, all Isese practitioners go to their shrines and make ose. To feed our orisas, we give offerings of specific foods and liquors. When giving offerings, we eat a small amount of the food and take a shot of *oti*, or liquor, after offering some to our shrines.

Through the process of making ose, we not only feed our shrines, we also feed ourselves. The meditative ritual of making ose feeds our spirits and nourishes the god within us, teaching us the practice of self-devotion. By connecting the worship of ourselves with the worship of the orisa, Ifá emphasizes the importance of internal divinity. Through this practice, we

cultivate our orí in preparation for the time in which we all become ancestors. Making ose is meant to be a meditative ritual and is treated as a time
to reflect on our goals and accomplishments while communing with the
orisas. Self-divinations can be performed by skilled aborisa to check in
with the orisas and ensure that all offerings have been accepted. The self-
reflection component of making ose encourages us to ground ourselves and
take stock of our lives on a frequent basis. Many spiritual practices encourage self-reflection, but the frequency in which Isese requires it means that
self-reflection is constantly on one's mind. Since we make ose every four
days, the time between each reflection is short.

UNDERSTANDING ÀÌKÚ

Longevity is a central component of Ifá, shaping the foundation of the practice. Often translated to mean immortality, *àìkú* is the Yoruba word for longevity. The root of *àìkú* is the word *iku,* meaning "death." When translated
directly, *àìkú* means "to avert death." Although this can be misconstrued
as meaning immortality, to avert death in the context of Isese Ifá means to
extend one's life so that death does not interrupt them on their path.

The key to longevity is flexibility. Karl Marx and Friedrich Engels
describe this in the context of dialectical materialism, a philosophical
approach to reality. It is the combination of dialectics and materialism and
provides the theoretical basis for Marxism. Dialectics is a method of rea-
soning that seeks to understand things concretely and fully, beyond their
appearance, and get to the deeper essence of the thing they are trying to
understand. For example, a dialectical perspective of ecology would be
understanding that the flora and fauna are interconnected, that their present forms have arisen from millions of years of evolution, and that they are
continuing to evolve. Dialectics leans into contradiction and understands
that the truth isn't objective; it's the full picture of varying ideas, experiences, and viewpoints.

Materialism is the idea that the material world has an objective reality
that is separate from the mind, that all thoughts are formed as a reaction to

experiencing the world around you. Ideas only arise as a result of material conditions. Thoughts are a reflection of matter that exists independently outside the mind. Materialism contrasts with idealism, which is the concept that the natural world adheres to ideas. Idealists follow a particular concept or framework, such as religion, and understand the world around them from that framing. Materialism recognizes that the material world is constantly changing, and therefore your thoughts and ideas adapt to that world. Idealism focuses on understanding the world through abstractions. Dogmatic religions are examples of idealism because they are rooted in a concept of the world and the universe that is unchanging and inflexible.

Ifá and the ADRs that branched off from it are much more flexible and fluid because of their materialist orientations. Ifá is often referred to as a non-faith-based tradition. Unlike Christianity, which requires worshippers to maintain faith in god, Ifá is a practice and tradition that is more focused on understanding the natural world than focusing on abstract religious concepts. It can be said that Ifá is a practice-based tradition, similar to Buddhism and Hinduism. There is a constant dialogue between humans and the natural world in the form of divination, herbalism, medicinal foods, spiritual baths, and more. Some common examples of this dialogue from other traditions include ayurveda, Indigenous American spiritual practices, and traditional Chinese medicine. What all of these practices have in common is deciphering information from the natural world to inform our physical, mental, and spiritual lives. Information gleaned from herbs, the seasons, foods, and animals provides a mirror for our inner selves. Since this information is highly interpretable, and these traditions are regionally specific, there is inherent flexibility within many traditional practices. Every practitioner will have a slightly different interpretation based on their material reality.

Longevity exists within the ancestral traditions that we continue to cultivate generation after generation. These traditions are passed down, altered, and modified over time to create a rich and dynamic culture. The ability to adapt traditions for the modern era is what keeps cultures alive. One of the oldest practices in the world is herbalism. Across cultures, understanding and communing with plants is a foundational component of life. Herbalism can be seen in the traditional dishes our families make, the material used to make traditional clothing, the oils we apply to our hair, and offerings we leave for our ancestors. As we've become more alienated from the supply chains that transport raw materials across the globe and the manufacturing and labor costs that turn those raw materials into products, it becomes easy to forget the central role plants and the natural world play in our lives.

The key to combating environmental alienation is to find creative ways to engage ourselves in the process of creation. By taking back control over how the products we use and the food we eat are created, we're able to reconnect to deep cultural and spiritual traditions by keeping them alive in the present. As I discuss later in the chapter, food sovereignty is a core way BIPOC communities are reconnecting with plant knowledge while taking control over how food is produced within their communities.

THE BASIS OF IFÁ IS HERBALISM

Herbalism is the central force behind Ifá and is thus one of the central ways that the principle of *àìkú* is brought to life. Like many indigenous cultural practices, herbalism plays a central role in every component of traditional Yoruba life. Ifá and other indigenous traditions are spiritual sciences that draw from the knowledge of plant medicine and with a deep spiritual understanding and reverence of nature. Indigenous spirituality is centered on a deep ancestral connection not just to the land but to the cosmos. It's about understanding one's place in the universe and using the world around you to develop a better understanding of how the universe works.

Ifá is a spiritual science built on the idea that the universe is composed of a large repository of information, and when deciphered via divination, that information can be used to change or alter one's destiny. The universe is in a state of constant creation. Òrúnmìlà is the witness to creation and an indispensable component of Ifá. As the husband of orisa Odu, Òrúnmìlà is the only orisa who knows all the destinies of everything in the universe. This is why we call upon Òrúnmìlà during divination and why the entire tradition is named after her husband: Odu refers to both the orisa and the cosmic archetypes that are said to be the children of her and Òrúnmìlà.

The core divination system within Ifá and its offshoots is based in a binary system, similar to the ways computers use binary code to encrypt data. The binary system in Ifá is used to decipher an odu, which provides an ancient understanding of different aspects of the universe. An odu can be thought of a mini universe that one can reside in at any given moment. Ifá is a spiritual matrix made up of multiple odus that act as cosmic archetypes that explain the organization of asé in the universe.[5] There are 256 odus, 16 of which are considered to be major odus. According to the tradition, orisa Odu and Ọ̀rúnmìlà gave birth to the 16 major odus, known as *olodu* ("owner of odu"). These odus are *meji,* or double odus. This means that each of the 8 sets of markings are identical. From these 16 major odus the remaining 240 odus were born. These secondary odus, known as ọmọ odu ("children of odu") contain some of the same characteristics as their parents but are distinct in their own right. They should not be thought of merely as a combination of their two parents but as unique individuals with their own set of characteristics and knowledge.[6]

Everyone is living within multiple odus at a time. There is an odu for the year that is deciphered at the beginning of the Yoruba calendar. There is an odu that is read shortly after a baby is born that determines the path they may take in life. Any time you seek guidance from a babalawo or iyanifa, a new odu will be deciphered to gain insight into the particulars of whatever it is you're experiencing and seeking. Each odu is determined through the process of divination using either ikin, sacred palm nuts, or an opele, a diviners chain. The divination process entails deciphering how the ikin or opele land on the opón ifá, the divination tray. After each toss of the ikin or opele, the babalawo or iyanifa will mark either one line or two parallel lines on the opón ifá. After sixteen throws, eight sets of markings either containing a single line or two parallel lines are drawn. The pattern born from these lines creates a specific odu.

Other types of divination in Ifá are obi divination and *merindilogun* or *diloggun* divination. Obi divination uses obi, four-lobe kola nuts, to divine. Diloggun divination uses sixteen cowrie shells. The type of divination used is determined by the experience of the practitioner. Only babalawos and iyanifas can use the sacred ikin or opele. Aborisas use obi to divine. At its core, Ifá is a spiritual system based on understanding the complementary forces of light and dark. Light and dark do not represent "good" and "evil"; in Ifá, light is expansion and dark is contraction. Ifá cosmology describes the universe as being created based on the interplay between expansion and contraction, light and dark. Light is considered a masculine force while dark is a feminine force. During divination, light is represented by one vertical line and dark by two vertical lines. These light and dark markings make up the symbols for each odu.[7]

The divination materials used in Ifá come from plants sacred to the Yoruba people. Palm nuts and kola nuts are two of the most sacred plants in Ifá. To consecrate a shrine, a special combination of herbs is used by babalawos and their apprentices. The exact herbs and sacred prayers that are used are hidden sacred knowledge. The secrecy of the tradition has helped in part to maintain its longevity. Typically, a concoction known as *omiero*, sacred water, is used to consecrate the sacred tools used in Ifá.[8] Omiero is made from a combination of sacred herbs, oils, water, and liquor. There are many different omiero concoctions used for different sacred rites within the tradition.

Osain (also spelled Osanyìn) is the orisa of plants and sacred knowledge. Together with Ọṣun, Osain has the power to both heal and harm through the combined powers within water and herbs. Osain is indispensable because of the central role herbalism plays within Ifá. Osain is said to be the owner of all *palos* (sticks) and is often used by babalawos to confer protection or to strengthen sacred tools. Herbs are also incorporated into the spiritual incense and soaps commonly used in Ifá to cleanse or attract a desired quality to the user. In place of spiritual soaps, ritual baths that incorporate specific omiero are used before certain ceremonies as a spiritual cleanse and to usher in health.

Much of my family's herbal knowledge was lost during the Second Great Migration. After my grandparents left their home in rural Alabama to move to South Los Angeles, they had little access to land and community. My grandmother's backyard garden allowed her to continue cultivating crops. She also tended to the garden in my parent's backyard, planting collard greens, hot peppers, and tomatoes. My parents focused on tending to the fruit trees that grew in their backyard. My favorite time of year was late spring, when the peach, plum, persimmon, and tangerine trees would be in full bloom, dusting our backyard with tiny pastel petals. Where possible, my family passed down the tradition of growing crops and tending to the land despite the urban and suburban environments we found ourselves in. We incorporated the fruit and vegetables we grew into the meals we cooked. We made lemonade from my grandmother Sandra's lemon tree and cooked collard greens and green beans from my grandmother Louise's garden. My early memories of growing food stayed with me into adulthood.

I spent a lot of time connecting to plant medicine during my time in Santa Barbara. The climate and culture there created an ideal environment for connecting with nature and exploring alternative healing modalities. I connected with community organizers at El Centro, a grassroots-led organization dedicated to working toward liberation for communities of color. El Centro's community garden, Somos Semillas, provided workshops for community members of all ages to learn about composting, planting, and harvesting. The garden was bursting with life. Medicinal plants like comfrey (*Symphytum officinale*), echinacea (*Echinacea purpurea*), and white sage (*Salvia apiana*) brought pollinators to the garden. We shared stories from our heritage about the plants we grew, combining knowledge from Chumash, Mexican, and African American herbalism. I attended community gatherings where we enjoyed home-cooked tamales and harvested corn and squash together. Learning from experienced farmers and herbalists allowed me to turn my herbal theory into praxis. It was an immensely rewarding experience to grow food for the community with the community. My life in Santa Barbara was made more beautiful by the time I spent in the community garden. I'm grateful for the friendships I made and the information I learned from Somos Semillas.

I use herbalism and plant medicine to stay grounded and connected to my own Ifá practice. Some of the ways I've discovered that help to keep myself grounded include cultivating herbs in my little apartment, growing mushrooms with my partner, spending time in community gardens, and making as many DIY products as I can. From teas, soaps, salves, *jun* (a beverage similar to kombucha but made with honey), and mead, I've seen how magical and transformative it is to take raw plant material and turn it into something tasty or useful. Herbalism and plant medicine are ways for us to connect to the ancestral; they're practices that root back into time, that our ancestors have used before us and that our descendants will use for generations to come.

One of the easiest ways to begin your own herbal practice is through cooking. Making dishes from scratch either from your culture or another invites you to explore and understand the ingredients in a new light. Look up recipes for *aguas frescas,* teas, stews, gumbos, and curries. Something as simple as making homemade lemonade can kick-start your journey into herbalism. If cooking isn't your thing, focus on a hobby or aspect of your daily routine that you cherish the most. If you're interested in skin care or hair care, you could begin by researching which herbs could improve skin texture and tone or increase hair health and shine. Herbs and oils like rosemary, hibiscus, turmeric, amla oil, and castor oil are known for their skin and hair health benefits. You might consider making your own hair oils or face masks as a way to familiarize yourself with the medicinal properties of plants.

If you're interested in music, you could begin by researching the materials used to make various instruments across different cultures and through time. For example, various gourds are used to craft instruments like the *shekere,* a percussive instrument made from a dried gourd and beads or cowrie shells. It is played across Africa and throughout the diaspora. You could also research the ways herbalism inspired or fueled musical creation in different ways. Many influential musicians took inspiration from psychedelic experiences ushered in by plant medicine. Timeless songs like Minnie Riperton's "Les Fleurs," Kali Uchis's recent album *Orquídeas,* Hiatus Kaiyote's song "Rose Water," and Joe Henderson's *Black Narcissus* album are some of my favorite examples of music inspired by the beauty of nature. Pick a plant (typically but not always a flower) and begin researching the music it inspired. Through this exploration, you'll discover how interconnected herbalism and plant knowledge are in our everyday lives, deepening your appreciation and reverence for the natural world around you.

Making my own herbal remedies is a meditative practice for me. It forces me to slow down and be patient. Plant medicine works on a different timeline than over-the-counter remedies. Making herbal remedies like tinctures and soaps can take weeks to months before they're ready to be used. I combine herbal knowledge from my family and herbalism books that focus on Black, Indigenous, and scientific herbalism. Combining knowledge from different perspectives creates a holistic approach to herbalism that honors ancestral wisdom and scientific knowledge.

African American herbal traditions incorporate a combination of the legacy of West African and Indigenous American herbal knowledge. When enslaved Africans were forcibly disconnected from their indigenous lands and transported to what is now known as the United States, they brought their knowledge of farming, their spiritual traditions, and their knowledge of plant medicine with them. Known for their skilled rice farming, enslaved Africans cultivated West African rice in the Americas, making the South incredibly wealthy. Carolina Gold refers to the rice cultivated in the region during slavery.[9] Along with rice, other herbs were brought from West Africa by both enslaved Africans and their captors. Indigo, black-eyed peas, and okra made their way to the Americas. Over time, enslaved Africans learned how to cultivate local plants, drawing from the existing wealth of Indigenous knowledge. Together, a rich culinary and spiritual culture was born from the unique ecological mixing within the Southern United States.

In *Working the Roots: Over 400 Years of Traditional African-American Healing,* Michele E. Lee explores the rich cultures and traditions of Black American herbalism. Through interviews with elders, Lee creates an archive of traditional healing modalities, folk wisdom, and ancestral knowledge. The vast plant medicine Lee expertly catalogs contains knowledge of plants native to the Americas, West Africa, and Europe. As I read through Lee's book, I discovered new herbal remedies and learned more information about the ones I had learned from my family. Castor oil, pot liquor, cayenne pepper, cow dung tea, cod liver oil, tallow, and walnuts were all connected to family stories. Most of these stories came from my mother recounting stories her mother and father had told her or recounting stories from her own childhood. My mother is not one to dabble in natural remedies, and although she didn't prescribe very many to me as a child, I learned a bit about them from her stories. I learned about my great uncle's farm where he grew a variety of vegetables, including peanuts that he would ship to my grandmother. I have memories of watching my grandmother roast her brother's peanuts in the oven while I sat on the floor shucking corn and peas that grew from her backyard garden. My mom told stories of her parents encouraging her and her sibling to take a spoonful of cod liver oil in the mornings as part of their daily routine. When my grandmother was young, her family sought out traditional healing remedies when Western medicine wasn't an option. My family, like many other Black families, struggled to access Western medicine due to systemic racism that excluded Black people from receiving medical care in many parts of the Deep South. Plant medicine served as an alternative to Western medicine, cultivating a sense of autonomy within Black communities. Plant medicine allowed Black people to care for themselves in ways that were both accessible and culturally relevant.

In her interview with Anita Poree, a Choctaw and Creole woman from Oklahoma, Mississippi, and Louisiana, Lee explores the unique ways herbalism intermixed with various spiritual traditions. Hailing from a multicultural background, Poree recounts her family's incorporation of Indigenous American, African, and European knowledge and how it influenced her identity today. Poree describes her spiritual beliefs as a blend of Indigenous American, Creole, Vodun, and Santería influences. Her approach to spirituality is rooted in a deep respect for nature and an understanding of plant medicine. Poree mixes and combines practices from various spiritual traditions. She incorporates the hoodoo practice of burning bay leaves with the Indigenous American practice of collecting cedar to purify and cleanse her space. Anita also talks about her family's practice of drinking pot liquor to improve their health. Pot liquor is the broth that's left after cooking a pot of greens. Drinking pot liquor is a common African American traditional medicine practice because of the vitamins and nutrients found in collard greens.[10]

INDIGENOUS AND ANCESTRAL PLANT MEDICINES

Held every year in South Carolina, the Gullah Geechee Herbal Gathering brings together Black herbalists throughout the region and across the nations for a conference aimed at uplifting Black and Indigenous herbal and spiritual wisdom. The goal of founder Khetnu Nefer, a certified doula and licensed massage therapist, was to provide a sacred space for Black and Indigenous healers, herbalists, hoodoo practitioners, and birth workers to gather, exchange ideas, and learn from people within their own communities. Workshops offered at the conference include incense making, yoga and meditation sessions, and various herbal workshops that deep-dive into specific plant medicines or treatments for specific ailments—workshops on herbal and nutritional interventions for diabetes, using flower essences to connect with ancestors, and hoodoo herbs for grief support.[11] The conference is often visited by Queen Quet, the elected chieftess of the Gullah Geechee Nation. Queen Quet advocates for the protection of Gullah lands from property developers and fights to preserve Gullah culture, traveling across the country and abroad to teach people about the history of the Gulla people. Vendors at the conference sell a variety of herbal products, merch, and handmade items, including traditional Gullah sweetgrass baskets. The baskets are made by weaving together sweetgrass and other plants like palm fronds in the tradition of West African basket weavers who carried their knowledge to the Americas during the transatlantic slave trade.

We often associate plant medicine with psychedelic or mood-altering experiences. Many indigenous communities around the world utilize the psychedelic effects of plant medicine for spiritual purposes. Since the 1970s, Americans have been fascinated in particular by the history of psychedelic plant medicine from Indigenous American communities in both North and South America. Spiritual tourism has led Westerners to travel throughout the Americas in search of psilocybin, peyote, and ayahuasca.

In recent years, Western tourism for psychedelic and mood-altering experiences has expanded to West-Central Africa. The Bantu-Kongo region encompasses the vast majority of Africa, stretching from West-Central Africa to South Africa and into the east. Within the region there are over four hundred different languages. The Bantu-Kongo region is also home to hundreds of distinct ethnic groups. Although diverse both ethnically and linguistically, there are some similarities between culture and religion among the Bantu-Kongo people. The Kongo region is composed of several

West-Central African nations including Gabon, the Democratic Republic of Congo, and Cameroon.

Primarily practiced in modern-day Gabon, Bwiti is a spiritual practice based in Kongo cosmology that's focused on healing the physical and spiritual body as well as the community. During initiation ceremonies, iboga, a psychoactive plant native to the region, is taken to help initiates build a deeper understanding of themselves and their place in their community through a hallucinogenic trance. Iboga (*Tabernanthe iboga*) contains the psychoactive compound called ibogaine, which is ingested by chewing the bark and root of the plant. The trance state that initiates enter after consuming iboga allows them to enter the spiritual realm of the ancestors. Iboga's ability to induce trance states has led to its association with the realm of the ancestors. Iboga is often described as a plant ancestor of the Bwiti devotees, indicating the deep connection of iboga within indigenous communities in Gabon.[12]

Cannabis is often incorporated in African healing and spiritual practices in West Africa and throughout the diaspora. In Gabon, *Cannabis sativa* is smoked during Bwiti initiation rituals to supplement the hallucinogenic effects of iboga. In Jamaica, cannabis is a core part of Rastafari spiritual practices. According to Rastafari cosmology, the "holy herb" mentioned in the Bible is a reference to cannabis, and the meditative state cannabis induced brings Rastafari practitioners closer to god. In the Caribbean, cannabis cultivation took off after indentured servants from India brought the plant with them. According to the Vedas, ancient Hindu text, *Cannabis sativa* is heralded as a divine plant.[13] The term *ganja* comes from the Hindi word for cannabis.

Despite the long history of cannabis within various indigenous communities and spiritual traditions, it remains a highly criminalized plant throughout many parts of the world. In the United States, cannabis legalization is handled on a state-by-state basis. Cannabis criminalization is responsible for the mass incarceration of Black and Latinx people in the United States. Though Black and white people sell and consume cannabis at roughly the same rate, Black people are four times more likely to be arrested for cannabis possession. In 2013 about thirteen thousand people were deported or separated from their communities due to cannabis possession.[14]

In parts of the country where cannabis possession and use is legalized, various organizations are working to heal some of the harm caused to Black and brown communities from cannabis criminalization. Black Bloom is a worker cooperative located in Los Angeles that provides free supplies and education to Black folks interested in learning how to grow their own cannabis flower at home. Through organic farming practices, Black Bloom centers Black farmers while building sustainable practices to support the future of cannabis growing and Black farming throughout the Los Angeles area.[15]

FOOD SOVEREIGNTY

Herbalism extends beyond understanding the medicinal and spiritual properties of plants. Learning how to grow and care for plants is a major part of deepening your herbal practice. Understanding how to grow your own food and medicine is a liberatory practice. It allows us to take back control over our health through sustainability and self-sufficiency. There are countless examples of Black people fighting for liberation through food. From farmers to spiritual leaders, Black people across the diaspora are using different approaches to food sovereignty to shape our communities.

The food sovereignty movement seeks to place the power and control over our food and agricultural systems in the hands of farmers and community members. At the 2007 convening at the first global International Forum on Food Sovereignty in Mali, over five hundred representatives from eighty countries created the Declaration of Nyéléni. The declaration defined food sovereignty as "the right of peoples to healthy and culturally appropriate food produced through ecologically sound and sustainable methods, and their right to define their own food and agriculture systems."[16]

Food sovereignty is a way to ensure that ancestral herbalism and farming practices are kept alive while also taking back control of the foods we consume. Many different BIPOC communities are focused on food sovereignty around the world. Food sovereignty practices include Indigenous seed keeping, maintaining traditional hunting practices, and urban farming. Food sovereignty embodies a core tenet in Ifá, which is the idea that there is no one correct path for everyone. Food sovereignty allows communities to build practices that are rooted in their unique cultural traditions while taking into account the ways larger systems of oppression have impacted them socially, economically, and health-wise.

Our current system of agribusiness creates ecological collapse by destroying the land and the soil. At least 30 percent of all greenhouse gas emissions come from the global food system.[17] Food sovereignty seeks to limit or remove ourselves from the global food system by focusing on local, culturally specific indigenous food systems and farming techniques. Food sovereignty is about the right for a people to determine their food agriculture policies for their communities rather than having their food supply subject to market forces and their land controlled by capitalist agribusinesses. Agroecology is a farming practice that incorporates indigenous knowledge into techniques that center on producing food without damaging natural resources. Access to healthy, culturally informed, and locally grown food is crucial to the health of Black and Indigenous communities.

West Africa

In West Africa, indigenous communities are approaching food sovereignty through agroecology. The Manjaque ethnic group lives in a peasant community south of the Cacheu River. Rice cultivation is the main agricultural practice and as a result is integral to community life. The Manjaques are a deeply spiritual community that relies on a variety of rice species not only for food but for traditional ceremonies like marriages, circumcisions, funerals, and rites of passage. Each event requires a different assortment of rice species. Recently, with imported broken rice, climate change, and less farming labor as young people move towns, the local rice cultivation has been threatened. To combat these threats, community members have held meetings across the region to share seed cultivation techniques, categorize and catalog the various seed species, and learn from elders. The result has been large-scale cultivation of all the wild rice seed varieties needed for traditional ceremonies in all the environmental zones (plateau, lowland, mangrove). The mobilization of young people in seed cultivation improved as elders shared community knowledge across environmental zones.[18]

In Benin, food security is threatened by agribusiness's overplanting of monocultures and irregular weather patterns. In the small village of Kom'dè, population 2,500, over 90 percent of the residents are food insecure. The Project for Adaptation to Climate Change (PAda-Clim-Benin) launched a family farm training program in agroecological practices focused on soil fertility, water conservation, and agroforestry using indigenous techniques. Through this program, crop yields have increased by 50 to 60 percent. Farmers report bigger yams, greater groundnut yields, and the return of previously lost crops like pigeon peas and soybeans.

East Africa

In East Africa, indigenous knowledge provides solutions to agricultural problems caused by climate change. Northern Ethiopia has historically been plagued by widespread long-term droughts that have led to starvation, death, and migrations in the region for centuries. However, in the mountainous regions of northern Ethiopia, some communities were able to maintain livestock and insulate themselves from the brunt of the drought's impact. *Ficus thonningii*, known locally as shibaka, is an evergreen tree species that is drought-resistant. Shibaka matures in one and a half to two years, prevents soil erosion, and supplies fodder for livestock year-round. Since 2006, a project initiated in Sefe'o village of Ahferom by Mekelle University's College of Dryland Agriculture and Natural Resources has trained farmers from over twenty thousand households in how to plant and maintain shibaka. The researchers measured the impact of shibaka on livelihoods, the environment, and climate change adaptations in both the traditional communities and the newly planted regions.[19]

The results of the decade-long data analysis are inspiring. *F. thonningii* leaves are incredibly nutrient-dense, with a protein content of 18 to 25 percent. *F. thonningii* leaves can replace costly commercial concentrates by up to 50 percent. As a result, cows produced twice as much milk per day compared to commercial feed. *F. thonningii* was able to improve physical and chemical indicators of soil quality and reduce water usage for livestock fodder by 85 percent. Farmers are now able to utilize previously arid land to raise successful livestock and shibaka. All of this was done at extremely low cost; *F. thonningii* is a tree indigenous to Ethiopia, making planting materials easily and readily available.

United States and the Americas

Food sovereignty among Black communities in the United States has taken on many different forms and is connected to many different yet interconnected social and political movements. Some of these movements include the Black veganism and plant-based eating movement, the Black farmers movement, the community garden and urban farming movement, the Black and queer ecology movement, the cannabis justice movement, and various Black spiritual movements. Each of these movements and communities are connected by a common thread: a desire to cultivate a deeper and more intentional relationship with plants. Each movement pursues this goal through different means, from advocating for protections for Black farmers to creating community spaces for BIPOC communities to practice plant medicine safely.

The violence of enslavement damaged our relationship to land. Although we've fought to maintain this relationship, many of us have trauma from the legacy of slavery, the history of sharecropping, and the loss of Black farmland. White farmers systemically pushed out Black farmers in the South, severed our ties to land, and reduced our ability to create autonomous communities. In 1910 about 14 percent of US farmers were Black, collectively owning 16 million acres of farmland. Today about 1 in 100 farmers are Black, equating to less than 5 million acres of farmland.[20] A large part of food sovereignty in Black American communities is focused on relearning and reestablishing our connection to the land. This includes starting our own farms, creating urban gardens, teaching young people about planting and harvesting, and talking to our elders about Black American plant medicines.

Soul Fire Farm. One of the leaders in the Black food sovereignty movement is Soul Fire Farm, based in Petersburgh, New York. Soul Fire Farm is an Afro-Indigenous-centered community farm dedicated to the goals of "uprooting racism and seeding sovereignty in the food system."[21] Through a combination of resources, including workshops, farmer training programs, and food distribution programs, Soul Fire Farm equips BIPOC communities with the tools and resources to build food sovereignty and resilience. Led by sisters Leah and Naima Penniman, Soul Fire Farm incorporates a variety of indigenous practices from around the world that inform their relationship to the land. In *Farming While Black*, Leah Penniman explores the topics of plant medicine, honoring the spirits of the land, and urban farming from an Afro-Jewish perspective. Throughout the book, Leah weaves in spiritual practices and traditions from her heritage that apply directly to reconnecting with the land and the natural. In the chapter "Raising Animals," Leah draws from both her Jewish and Black heritage, incorporating Hebrew, Vodou, and Yoruba prayers for the transition of life and to honor death during the process of animal slaughter.[22] In the chapter "Plant Medicine," Leah shares the geographic origins of common herbs like ashwagandha *(Withania somnifera)*, wormwood *(Artemisia absinthium)*, and hibiscus *(Hibiscus sabdariffa)*. She also includes information about how to process plant medicine by making salves, tinctures, baths, and oils.

Black Oregon Land Trust. Founded and led by a team of Black women and femmes, the Black Oregon Land Trust (BOLT) works to eliminate the barriers that prevent Black families from accessing the land. BOLT is rooted in a land sovereignty–centered approach that is focused on food justice and cultural preservation.[23] Three pillars make up the conceptual framework for BOLT's farm and community work. The first pillar is land access and preservation. Through their trust, BOLT transfers land stewardship to Black farmers in Oregon to ensure that future generations have access to land, food, housing, and community. Through the implementation of ancestral agricultural practices, BOLT aims to tend to and restore the land rather than deplete it. The second pillar is farming and food justice, aimed at building sustainable food systems by improving access to land ownership, mentorship, and training for Black farmers. The last pillar of cultural sovereignty focused on reclaiming ancestral ways of connecting to the land prior to colonization. Through each of these three pillars, BOLT provides space for Black farmers to access land and reconnect with traditional practices rooted in sustainability to build a robust agricultural system for generations to come.

Compton Community Garden. For over a decade, the Compton Community Garden has provided fresh produce, community gathering space, and agricultural classes to the South Los Angeles community. In April 2023 the community garden was threatened when a "For Sale" sign suddenly appeared on the property. The property owner listed the garden plot for sale without consulting the community garden. In a little over a month, the Compton Community Garden rallied the local community and successfully raised over $600,000 to counter the existing bid on the property.[24] The Compton Community Garden continues to provide community workshops on composting and organic gardening, carving out a space for Black urban farmers and community members to gather.

Crop Swap LA. An urban farming initiative founded by Jamiah Hargins in 2018, Crop Swap LA has grown into an urban farming movement that addresses food insecurity in South Los Angeles by turning underused spaces into urban microfarms across the city. Crop Swap LA grows a variety of foods suited to urban environments. Leafy greens, herbs, and root vegetables are selected for their short growing cycles and their suitability for farming in small spaces. Their urban farming workshop series aims to reduce food insecurity by educating the community on urban farming practices that lead to increased resiliency.[25]

Rastafari Ital Food. Food sovereignty within the Caribbean takes many forms. In Jamaica and the surrounding regions, some practitioners of Rastafari, a religious and political movement founded in Jamaica in the 1930s, eat a vegetarian diet known as ital. Derived from the word *vital,* ital is a diet tradition that focuses on increasing one's liveliness and longevity. Ital cuisine places an emphasis on one's spiritual connection to the food and the land. Food is vegetarian and free from processed foods and additives. Flavor is added by primarily using herbs and spices rather than salt, since many salt products are artificially modified. When possible, kosher salt and sea salt are used as a replacement for table salt.[26]

When I went to Jamaica in 2022, I visited Prapa Spice, a vegan food stall that sells hot made-to-order ital food in Montego Bay. I ordered a plate of chickpea curry, yam, and lentil stew on top of a bed of quinoa. I was blown away by how comforting and familiar the flavors were. I left inspired to incorporate ital recipes into my own plant-based cooking back home. Through culinary and spiritual culture, Prapa Spice approaches food sovereignty by cooking healthy meals for the community.

Finca Conciencia. The first agroecology farm on the island of Vieques, off the coast of Puerto Rico, Finca Conciencia is run by Ana Elisa Pérez Quintero and Jorge Cora. The 8.5-acre farm provides fresh, local produce to Vieques's ten thousand residents. Through growing vegetables, beekeeping, hosting workshops, and saving seeds, Pérez Quintero and Cora hope to build a food sovereignty movement on the island. Food sovereignty is a major issue in Puerto Rico, where 85 percent of food is imported. On Vieques, where food is transported to the island using an unreliable ferry system, food insecurity is an even bigger issue.[27]

Vieques has also experienced several environmental catastrophes. For six decades, the US Navy used Vieques as a weapons testing site, turning half the island into a Superfund site, recognized by the US Environmental Protection Agency as containing high amounts of hazardous and toxic waste.

Cora's work beekeeping on Vieques is crucial to the ecological sustainability of Puerto Rico. After 2017's Hurricane Maria, 80 percent of Puerto Rico's bee colonies were wiped out. Together, Cora and Pérez Quintero formed the collective La Colmena Cimarrona to teach agroecology workshops on beekeeping, composting, seed keeping, and a variety of other farming techniques. Their approach to farming is rooted in knowledge from the Taíno, the Indigenous people of the Caribbean. Through their farm, Pérez Quintero and Cora hope to build a sustainable food system based in Indigenous wisdom for Vieques while also working to combat displacement, gentrification, and land speculation.

Lakou Dantes is an Afro-Indigenous healing quilombo and sacred herbal farm in Jacmel, Haiti. *Quilombo* was originally a term used to describe communities formed by Black people who escaped enslavement, similar to a maroon community. Lakou Dantes embodies the spirit of fugitive slave communities by creating a space rooted in experimentation, ancestral traditions, and autonomy.[28] Founded by Manbo Lanise Colon, Lakou Dantes is a collective of healers, *mambos* (Haitian Vodou priestesses), and *oungans*

(Haitian Vodou priests) working with "lwa and ancestors to steward sacred land." Core to Lakou Dantes philosophy is the importance of spiritual intervention in community healing. Their offerings include a mix of spiritual rituals and traditional healing practices such as doula care, spiritual baths, and bone and curio divination. Immersed in everything at Lakou Dantes is a reverence for the land, the ancestors, and Haitian Vodou.

CONCLUSION

Our ancestors carried their knowledge about agriculture and plant medicine with them across the Atlantic. Informed by the spiritual traditions of West and West-Central Africa, the wisdom our ancestors brought with them created a spiritual science based in a deep understanding of the mind, body, and spirit. They studied the world around them and created an agricultural body of knowledge that incorporates African and Indigenous science. Their spiritual traditions, rooted in an understanding of nature, informed their philosophical approach to the land. They understood that land was sacred and to be respected. Land was shared communally among community members and relatives.

Our ancestors believed that everything has a spiritual energy. The key to any healing practice is to understand the medicinal and spiritual properties of plants. Spiritual practices like Ifá teach us how to be in relationship with nature. Worshipping the orisa teaches us to approach nature with humility and respect. The earth is our oldest teacher. Too often humans forget that we are one of the youngest species on the planet. We delude ourselves into thinking we are the highest form of intelligence and that we have everything figured out. There's so much we can learn from studying how the forces of nature interact with each other. The orisa are our ancestors; the interplay between them gave birth to life on earth. When we reframe our perspective to think about the forces of nature as our relatives, we remind ourselves of the interconnectedness of ecological systems and our place within them.

West African spiritual understandings that come from practices like Ifá and the Kongo cosmogram are based in cycles of rebirth. Everything in nature follows cycles of birth, death, and rebirth. The changing of the seasons and the cycles of the moon remind us that the universe is iterative in nature. The separation between birth and death, this world and the next, is a thin veil. Nothing that leaves us is ever truly gone. Our ancestors live on within us, in our memories and in our DNA. Communication with our elders and ancestors is crucial to our survival. The challenges they faced in their lifetime will reemerge in ours and in future generations. We can learn from their ingenuity to help us navigate the challenges we face in the future.

Retracing my family's history from Los Angeles to Alabama, Louisiana, and South Carolina has helped me piece together a narrative that brings me closer to understanding my family's place in Black history. Situating my mother's stories about our family's traditional healing practices within the larger context of African American healing traditions has added context to my grandparents' lives. These traditions were passed down by word of mouth, from one generation to the next. Like many other Black American families, my family abandoned their traditional healing practices during the Great Migration. Without access to land, it was difficult for Black families to continue the traditions of their ancestors. A lot of families also felt that the traditional wisdom from their elders was superstitious, backward, and outdated. A few generations later, many Black people across the diaspora are reclaiming their traditions. Taking knowledge from our ancestors and elders, younger generations are addressing the violence of food insecurity, displacement, and environmental racism by creating urban farms and land trusts.

African American and African diasporan healing practices were essential to our ancestors' survival during slavery, colonization, and Jim Crow. I feel honored to carry on the torch by investigating the techniques my ancestors used to survive and reimagining them for today. Black people still struggle to survive amid the racism and anti-Blackness inherent in our capitalistic and extractionist systems. To survive, we must find ways to heal our mind, body, and spirit. Healing our mind begins with decolonizing our worldview and reframing our ancestral knowledge as Afro-Indigenous science, not superstitious folly. When we recognize and affirm the intelligence of our ancestors, we affirm our cultural traditions as a whole. We can combine their understanding of plant medicine with a modern scientific under-standing to create healing practices that are culturally informed to heal our bodies. Healing our spirit requires us to heal our trauma associated with the land and find new ways to connect to nature that speak to us. We have to investigate the stories of our ancestors within our own families, digging up buried traditions and uncovering secrets that bring us closer to under-standing who we are. We can learn from our collective ancestors across the diaspora to fill in the missing pieces. When we combine the wisdom of our collective histories, we're able to reimagine new ways to heal and support our community as we continue on the path toward liberation.

2

THE BLESSING OF ÀJÉ

Why is it that the modern world can't deal with its
ancestors and endure its past?
—MALIDOMA PATRICE SOMÉ, *OF WATER AND THE SPIRIT*

When we think of wealth, our thoughts tend to center on monetary value. Money, power, capitalism, legacy, accumulation, scarcity. Wealth as we know it is an illusive and fickle force that we spend our entire lives in the pursuit of. Wealth is so integral to our lives as people living within a capitalistic system that an entire economy exists around teaching people how to acquire it. Colleges and universities promise that by investing tens of thousands of dollars in their programs, you will be able to secure wealth by first securing a job. From career centers and résumé workshops, academic institutions attempt to gamify the process. If you change the font on your résumé or use a different set of keywords, that will surely be your ticket into the high-paying career of your dreams. Social media influencers promising a fast track to wealth through cryptocurrency, investments, drop shipping, multilevel marketing schemes, real estate, monetization, and credit card hacks are more popular than ever. It seems like everyone on social media has figured out *the* way to acquire wealth. If you just pay for their online course, you too can have access to a six-figure income from the comfort of your bedroom.

Wealth is something I've fixated on to varying degrees throughout my life. Growing up in Orange County, monetary wealth provided you with social capital and allowed you to move through spaces with ease. My parents were well off and had the ability to buy me the latest fashion. But just because they had the ability to didn't mean they always did. There was a constant competitiveness among both the children and adults in my community. I understood from a very young age that within my hometown, wealth was the fastest ticket to "building community."

My idea of community was warped because it was connected to wealth. I grew up with messaging that told me to focus on superficial and materialistic aspects of people rather than focus on building deep and meaningful relationships from common interests and goals. Wealth and the pursuit of wealth warps our perspective and shapes the way we relate to each other. It degrades deep and meaningful connection in favor of superficial relationships predicated on status. Real community building comes from valuing the cultural, intellectual, and spiritual wealth gained from collaborating with other people.

THE CONCEPT OF WEALTH IN IFÁ

Àjé is the orisa of wealth, prosperity, and abundance. Personified as a feminine entity, Àjé is often associated with the deep ocean and birds, and she is one of the most illusive and lesser-known orisas. Though Àjé survived the transatlantic slave trade and was incorporated into Lukumi in the Americas, she did not become as well-known as other orisas like Ọṣun and Ṣàngó. Àjé is known for her shapeshifting ability, making her an orisa that is difficult to pin down and hard to fully understand. We can demystify Àjé by breaking apart the word into its core components to decipher the deeper meaning behind the spirit of wealth, prosperity, and abundance. In Yoruba, the prefix *à-* is a "noun maker," directly translating to "the one who." The suffix *-jé* translates to "the one who allows or causes; becomes; answers, responds, or works." These translations give way to multiple meanings for Àjé, which include "the one who allows or causes," "the one who becomes," and "the one who answers, responds, or works."[1] Àjé as "the one who becomes" speaks to the transformational power of wealth and abundance.

Wealth in Ifá is conceptualized beyond monetary gains and materialistic accumulation. Since abundance is a foundational concept in Ifá, wealth is not necessarily something to be sought after. Within a framework of abundance, Ifá teaches us that we already have more than enough. Everything we need has been selflessly gifted to us by Iya Aye, Mother Earth. Nature is the manifestation of the wealth and prosperity that surrounds us, and by focusing on the longevity of our traditions and practices, we are able to maintain the abundance nature has to offer us across generations. Before Ire Àjé, the blessings of wealth and prosperity, can be actualized, you must first focus on Ire Àìkú, the blessing of longevity. Utilizing a system that withstands the test of time and draws from knowledge from past generations to help inform future generations creates a foundation and framework for how to cultivate the other four blessings in Ifá.

Longevity and wealth are conceptualized as legacy within the context of Ifá. Legacy in Ifá cosmology is built through your impact in your community and is carried on by your children, family, or ilé. For Ifá to survive, spiritual leaders had to build communities that would continue to honor them and their teachings after their death. Ifá is built on ancestral knowledge that was passed down from generation to generation for thousands of years. That sacred information was then carried to the Americas and translated into several different languages. Ifá has transformed over time, drawing from Christian and Catholic traditions, incorporating modern gender theory, and finding a home for itself on the internet. Our ancestors' legacy can be felt through the cultural traditions that have been painstakingly cultivated and maintained by dedicated practitioners around the world. Wealth in Ifá is about the strength of your community, the legacy of your culture, and the richness of your traditions.

BLACK CAPITALISM AND WESTERN CONCEPTS OF WEALTH

Capitalism, the very force that has warped our perception of wealth, is also the force that attempted to eradicate Afro-Indigenous traditions. Capitalism is so deeply ingrained in the West that it's hard to imagine a world without it. Since capitalism is such a central concept in the American psyche, it's no wonder that the myth of Black capitalism has been so persistent. Living in a world that revolves around money impacts the ways we relate to each other. We begin to think in terms of scarcity and competition rather than abundance and community. When capitalism is the dominant ideology, people begin to believe that the only way we can support our communities is through the acquisition of monetary wealth. By acquiring monetary wealth, people believe that some of it will eventually "trickle down" into the community. This is the foundation of Black capitalism, the belief that by uplifting Black wealth, the entire Black community will benefit. When you operate in a scarcity mindset, it becomes difficult to think that you have enough. Wealth is acquired through the process of hoarding resources and capital. Only a minuscule amount of those hoarded resources will be redistributed to the community if the goal is to achieve monetary wealth and status.

Capitalism as an economic ideology traces its early roots to the transatlantic slave trade and the colonization of West Africa. In *How Europe Underdeveloped Africa,* Walter Rodney breaks down the way capitalism was used as a tool to lead to the economic underdevelopment of Africa through the conquest of land and people for the sake of profit. Rodney explains how religion is a core component of the economic structure of a society. Through the process of battling with a materialist environment, humans created various forms of social relations, government, patterns of behavior, and systems of belief that were unique from one another. This collection of societal components is what Rodney refers to as the "superstructure" of a society. Belief in an indigenous spiritual tradition that is rooted in reverence for nature tends to create societies that are structured communally. Rodney states that "the religious belief that a certain forest was sacred was the kind of element in the superstructure that affected economic activity, since that forest would not be cleared for cultivation."[2]

Nature-based traditions acted as a protective mechanism against capitalism and imperialism. Although all human societies cultivated the land for production, there were limits to the extent of that production based on the spiritual and communal beliefs of any given community. In Isese Ifá and other West African belief systems, the iroko tree (*Milicia excelsa*) is considered sacred and represents the connection between the physical world and the ancestral world, with the spirit of egúngún dwelling inside. Cutting down an iroko tree without permission from the spirit of the tree or the ancestors is believed to bring misfortune. In Haiti, the *mapou* tree (*Cyphostemma mappia*) serves a similar spiritual function in Haitian Vodou.[3] Beliefs rooted in the sacredness of nature act as a protective element against overconsumption.

Capitalism sits at the heart of colonialism. In *Discourse on Colonialism*, Aimé Césaire examines the origins of colonization and its relationship with Christianity. In his analysis, Césaire gets to the root of what drives colonization, claiming that it is not "evangelization, nor a desire to push back the frontiers of ignorance, disease, and tyranny, nor a project undertaken for the greater glory of god, nor an attempt to extend the rule of law." Religion is often used as a tool to advance colonial and capitalist projects by providing a "divine" explanation for the atrocities of colonization. To Césaire, colonization is driven by the desire to advance economically by any means necessary. He identifies the key actors in colonization as "the adventurer and the pirate, the wholesale grocer and the ship owner, the gold digger and the merchant, appetite and force." Césaire argues that behind these key actors is "the baleful shadow of a form of civilization which, at a certain point in its history, finds itself obliged, for internal reasons, to extend to a world scale the competition of its antagonistic economies."[4] To seek new markets and increase capital gains, capitalism demands expansion into new territories in search of new goods, labor, and consumers. Colonialism is the result of an economic philosophy grounded in expansionism and profit. To maximize profit, cheap labor in the form of serfdom, slave labor, and indentured servitude was foundational to the growth of the European economy and the economy of Europe's colonies. In search of cheap labor and goods and resources to sell, colonizers invaded nations around the world. By toppling governments, destroying existing economies, and enslaving Black and Indigenous people, Europe seized the natural resources of Africa and the Americas and used cheap labor to fuel their economic growth.

In *The Nation on No Map: Black Anarchism and Abolition*, William C. Anderson discusses the connection between wealth and the mythologies surrounding Black ancestry. Capitalism infects our minds and movements, limiting our imaginations and restricting our worldview. The desire to be wealthy poses a barrier to collective liberation. Despite understanding the limitations of capitalism, many people still desire to be in proximity to wealth and celebrity. As the descendants of enslaved Africans, Black people often long to know more about their ancestry and to connect to a past that was violently stripped from them. In an attempt at reconnection, some people create mythologies about Black ancestry and history that mirror the capitalist values of the West. Mythologies about Egypt or that uphold monarchs like Emperor Haile Selassie of Ethiopia are rooted in a desire to prioritize stories about African royalty over the lives of the everyday Africans we descend from. Anderson explains that emphasizing African royalty as a sense of pride "reproduces the notion that wealth and power is what determines a person's value."[5] Uplifting African royalty creates false narratives about our ancestry and idolizes systems of oppression that replicate the violent oppression Black people experience in the diaspora.

Egypt is commonly idolized as the pinnacle of African empire building. Black diasporans have attempted to lay claim to Egypt by fabricating false identities rooted in Egyptian ancestry or supposed Egyptian practices. Reaching to East Africa as a source of connection for Black diasporans flattens the African continent in the same ways the West homogenizes Africa. The homogenization of Africa, which reduces the continent to a "country" in the Western imagination, ignores the geographic and cultural magnitude of Africa. Africa is the second-largest continent, accounting for one-fifth of the earth's land mass.[6] Egypt and Nigeria exist on opposite sides of the continent. Though there are clear similarities between African cultures across the continent, Egypt's influence on West Africa is minimal.

The same argument can be made when discussing Christianity in Africa. Christianity's influence in West Africa and throughout the African diaspora is directly connected to capitalism. Through the capitalist conquest of the transatlantic slave trade and the colonization of Africa, Christian missionaries converted Africans on the continent and in the Americas. Rather than acknowledge the vast religious diversity that exists among the hundreds of tribal and ethnic groups that make up the African continent, some Black diasporans justify Christianity's presence in West African and African diasporic life because of its early presence in Ethiopia and other parts of East Africa.

The descendants of enslaved Africans who want to create a past they are proud of through mythologies that forget about "the distinctions between the rulers and the ruled."[7] In reimagining ourselves as the kings and queens of Africa, we forget many African rulers facilitated the very slave trade that stripped us of our homeland. There's a danger in forgetting the role African rulers played in the transatlantic slave trade. When we forget the complex history of colonization and enslavement, we risk creating another type of mythology rooted in the belief that Black and Indigenous peoples are not capable of replicating the violent forces of colonization, genocide, and enslavement. The mythology that exists within a particular community has the power to become a dangerous force when it begins to disconnect people from a sense of community grounded in the belief that all life is sacred and worthy of protection. In idolizing Christianity's presence in Ethiopia, we ignore the violence of colonialism and the role Christianity played in the slave trade. So long as we aspire to replicate whiteness and seek Western markers of success, we will continue to replicate the same violence in our communities.

LOSS AND TRANSFORMATION OF COMMUNITY

In 1483 the Portuguese arrived in the Kongo Kingdom. By 1491, King Nzinga a Nkuwu and his son were baptized by the Catholic Church. Their baptism was symbolic of the alliance formed between the Kongo Kingdom and Portugal. Enslaved Africans already existed prior to the arrival of the Portuguese. The Kongo slave trade was relatively small, didn't typically enslave women, and didn't enslave Kongolese subjects. The Portuguese disrupted the indigenous slave trade and implemented their own, destabilizing the Kongo Kingdom in the process. King Afonso's rise to power in 1506 began the centuries-long campaign against indigenous Kongo traditions. Afonso was a devout Christian who worked tirelessly to rid his kingdom of "idolaters" and "infidels." By 1619, when the first enslaved Africans reached the British colonies that would become the United States, many of them were Christian Africans from Kongo.[8]

The origins of Christianity among West Africans and the descendants of West Africans is a violent one that is intricately tied to capitalism. In her book *Lose Your Mother*, Saidiya Hartman recounts her journey to Ghana as a Black woman raised in the United States who is attempting to reconnect with her "lost" heritage. Throughout the book Saidiya weaves in stories of her own experience in Ghana with the political forces that shaped Ghana shortly after gaining independence from Britain and the history of enslavement on the West African coast. Hartman recounts the violence of Christianity and capitalism through her examination of slave ports along the Gold Coast of Africa. Many of the people taken from Benin and sold into enslavement were women and girls between the ages of ten and twenty; in the 1540s, the *oba*, the ruler or king, of Benin attempted to curb the sale of men and boys, eventually attempting to prohibit it altogether. Upon capture, young women and girls were branded with a cross on their arms or breasts. They were then transported on slave ships bearing names like *Christ the Redeemer, Amistad, Blessed, John Evangelist, The Lord Our Savior, Recovery,* and *Trinity*.[9] To say that Christianity, capitalism, and enslavement are not deeply intertwined would be a gross misrepresentation of history.

Through the violent process of enslavement, enslaved Africans had their identities and cultures stripped from them. Hartman describes the ways entire communities were decimated by the transatlantic slave trade. Among the people captured in Kongo, Hartman describes them as "prisoners of war taken by marauding armies; artisans, farmers, healers, weavers, fishermen, and metalworkers captured in raids on their towns and villages; undesirables, criminals, and troublemakers sentenced to slavery; and students, the sons of Kongolese nobles, kidnapped in São Tomé on their journey to seminary in Lisbon."[10]

People from all walks of life were stripped of their identity in the process of enslavement. A "slave" is a fictitious identity that is created through a complex process of dehumanization through violence. To Hartman, "the dungeon was the womb in which the slave was born." She argues that "slavery made your mother into a myth, banished your father's name, and exiled your siblings to the far corners of the earth."

While the Middle Passage destroyed identities, it simultaneously birthed a new one. This new identity was "an identity produced by negation."[11] The immense loss of language, trades, cultures, traditions, and economies shapes African diasporic experiences. It is an inevitable and deliberate artifact of the immense violence of enslavement. Stripping people of their identity makes them easier to control and subjugate. When you don't know where you came from, it becomes difficult to see where you are going.

ATRs IN THE AMERICAS

Despite the violent attempts to eradicate African cultures, enslaved Africans managed to hold on to their traditions and practices by transforming and adapting them to new environments. Through the process of cultural adaptation, new and rich practices developed that incorporated Afro-Indigenous wisdom, Indigenous plant knowledge, and European customs. These practices are just as valid as traditions on the African continent. West Africa is just as impacted by the legacy of enslavement as Africans living in the diaspora. From gross mistranslations of indigenous languages to the widespread adoption of Christianity, West African customs and traditions have been forever altered by the transatlantic slave trade. Hartman describes many of the people she met in Ghana as similar to many African Americans in terms of their perspectives on aesthetics, religion, and political ideology. She claims that "it was ironic that the kind of African Americans who would fit best in Ghana were the ones least attracted to Africa. The straightened-hair, prim, Bible-thumping, flag-waving Black Christian conservatives would be much more at home in Ghana than the frayed band of dreadlocked and nappy-headed radicals who inundated the place. Evangelicals were welcome; protestors need not apply."[12] The impact of colonization can be felt among all African peoples, and it's important to remember this when talking about the validity of Black cultural traditions and practices. For the purpose of survival, African diasporic traditions had to change and transform, as did traditions within the African continent. Cultures are living things that grow and change over time.

Adechina is one of the figures who will help us understand the connection between West African traditions and those that exist within the diaspora. Adechina, also known as Ño Remigio Herrera Adeshina Obara Meji, was a babalawo from the Oyo kingdom in modern-day Nigeria who is credited as one of the key people who brought Ifá to Cuba in the early 1800s. Not much information is known about his early life in Nigeria. Sometime in the early 1800s, Adechina was captured by enslavers and brought to Cuba. News of the arrival of slave traders had spread throughout Adechina's community. Prior to being captured, Adechina swallowed his ikin (sacred palm nuts) in order to smuggle them with him.

Adechina arrived in Cuba in the late 1820s and was given the name Remigio Herrara. It is unknown how long Adechina worked on his owners' plantation and what his relationships were with the other enslaved Africans. Over time he gained the trust of his plantation owners. They enlisted him to run errands on their behalf, permitting him to travel between plantations. It was on one of these trips that he met Adé Bí, another babalawo from Nigeria who was enslaved. Adé Bí managed to gain the trust of his enslavers by performing divination to help them with their financial affairs. With the help of Adé Bí, Adechina managed to clean and feed his ikin that he had kept hidden from his plantation owners. Once the ikin are cleaned and fed, they're able to be used for divination. Adechina began divining for his community, earning him recognition. After several years, with the help of his community, Adechina was able to buy his freedom. He went on to start a *cabildo de nación*, a type of ethnic council that functioned as secret societies among freed Africans in Cuba. Throughout his lifetime, Adechina became a leader in his community, providing spiritual services and leading initiation ceremonies. Adechina was one of many babalawos that was transported to the Americas during the slave trade. Through his work, and the work of others like him, African spiritual practices were preserved in Cuba and across the diaspora.[13]

Adechina and other enslaved Africans created ADRs like Lukumi, Winti, Candomblé, and hoodoo. African traditions vary widely throughout the diaspora. Some take the form of structured traditions with an organized set of rituals and taboos. Others are less structured, typically consisting of a collection of folk traditions that are incorporated into medical and spiritual practices.

Lukumi, Santería, Regla de Ocha

Lukumi, also known as Santería or Regla de Ocha, is the Yoruba-based spiritual practice developed by enslaved Africans in Cuba. Lukumi resembles Isese Ifá in many ways, from the language to the ceremonial rituals, and they are closely related. Lukumi, also spelled Lucumi, refers to both the spiritual tradition and the language. In both Isese and Lukumi, the practitioners speak Yoruba or a "creoled" version of Yoruba when singing songs or speaking ritualistic prayers. Lukumi is the Hispanicized or Latinized Yoruba dialect spoken by devotees of the tradition. When Ifá took root in Cuba, the names of the orisa, songs, and prayers were retained. Over time the pronunciations and spellings changed, and in some cases new names were used to describe elements of the tradition. An example is the different names and pronunciations for the orisa Esu. Esu is often referred to as Elégbà in Yoruba or Elegua in Lukumi. Lukumi priests are called babalawos, *santeros,* or *padrinos.* They perform the same functions as babalawos in Isese Ifá.

Key differences exist between Isese and Lukumi, particularly around each tradition's rituals relating to shrines. Isese tends to focus on the cultivation of an Ifá shrine known as one's Hand of Ifá. Lukumi focuses on receiving one's *guerreros,* or warriors. The warriors consist of individual shrines for Esu, Ògún, Ochoosi, and Ọṣun, each consecrated by a babalawo.[14]

Yoruba spiritual practices are not dogmatic and don't require devotees to exclusively adhere to the Yoruba spiritual system. This allowed enslaved Africans in Cuba to mix several different traditions together, sometimes incorporating Roman Catholic iconography into the tradition.

Candomblé and Umbanda

Candomblé and Umbanda are the Yoruba-based spiritual traditions practiced in Brazil that incorporate some Roman Catholic practices, much like Santería. The structure of Candomblé and Umbanda closely mirrors that of

Lukumi and Isese and similarly requires practitioners to follow the practices of their particular *terrerio,* or spiritual house. Candomblé priests are
referred to as *babalaxe* and priestesses are *yialaxe.*

Palo Mayombe

Throughout the diaspora, Lukumi and Palo Mayombe are often practiced
together. Lukumi and Palo operate as sister traditions. It's common for
people to be initiated in both and to use techniques from each for different
purposes. Palo Mayombe, also known as Las Reglas de Congo, is a spiritual practice based in rituals and traditions from Kongo. *Palo,* Spanish for
"stick," refers to the spiritual presence found in herbs. Like other ATRs and
ADRs, herbs are a central component in Palo Mayombe rituals.

The essence of Palo Mayombe is the *nganga.* In Kongo, an nganga is a
priest trained in medicinal and spiritual knowledge, similar to a babalawo
among the Yoruba in Nigeria. In Palo, an nganga is a large clay pot or iron
cauldron filled with items containing spiritual power and ritualistic significance. The contents of the nganga are used to strengthen the connection
to the ancestral realm and to the earth.[15] Contents of ngangas can include
bones, candles, and wooden stakes called palos. Similarly to a shrine in
Isese or Lukumi, the nganga serves as the physical epicenter for a particular
spiritual entity or force.

In Palo Mayombe, the spirits of the natural world are called *mpungus.*
Nsai (spirit of fire and lightning), Sarabanda (spirit of war and iron), and
Baluandé (spirit of water, motherhood, and fertility) are three common
mpungus that serve as the Palo counterparts to Ṣàngó, Ògún, and Yemayá,
respectively.[16] Priests who've undergone initiation and are trained in spiritual matters are referred to as *paleros,* and they perform ceremonies and
conduct initiations. Before initiation, the initiate undergoes a ritual bath or
cleansing known as a *limpieza* or *omiero. Limpieza* or *limpia* is also a term
used to describe Afro-Latin cleansing rituals more broadly. These rituals
are based in Indigenous American practices for cleansing and purification.[17]
A common limpia called *limpia con huevo* involves rubbing an egg all over
the body to remove negative energy before cracking it in a glass of water to
"read" the egg. *Omiero* is the Yoruba term for "sacred herbal water" and is a

type of spiritual bath used to remove negative energy. The use of both limp-ieza and omiero in Palo illustrate the ways different Indigenous and Yoruba cultural practices influence the tradition.

During a Palo Mayombe initiation, the initiate receives several cut marks on key points on the body. Undergoing initiation into Palo is called being "scratched." *Firmas*, elaborate symbols drawn to connect to the mpungu, are drawn on the ground to contact the spiritual forces required for the initiation process.

Haitian Vodou

Vodou contains many of the same spiritual elements found in Ifá and Kongo cosmology. Vodou is connected to spiritual practices from the Fon and Ewe people of mondern-day Benin and the Yoruba of Nigeria and Benin.[18] Vodou centers on the belief in a supreme creator, referred to as Bon Dieu (Kreyol: Bondye) and Grand Maître (Kreyol: Gran Mèt), and spirits know as lwa or loa. Similarly to Olódùmarè, Bon Dieu is a distant creator that does not directly interact with humans. Through the lwa, which represent different aspects of Bon Dieu, devotees are able to communicate with the spiritual realm. The lwa represent the forces of nature and share many commonalities with Yoruba orisa. Esu, Obatala, Ògún, and several other orisas have counterparts in Vodou. The Vodou pantheon also consists of lwa unique to the tradition, such as Damballah or Dambala Ouedo, "the supreme Mystere and his signature is the serpent."[19] Damballa is one of the most important lwa. He represents creation and rebirth and is closely associated with snakes.

Veves, a symbol drawn to invoke the lwa, are similar in both form and function to firmas in Palo Mayombe. Veves are a central component of Haitian Vodou, the spiritual tradition born from West African practices. A Vodou priest is referred to as a *hougan* or *oungan* and a priestess as a *manbo* or *mambo*.[20]

Voodoo, Hoodoo, Rootwork, and Conjure

Voodoo in the United States, though influenced by Haiti, is a completely different practice. In the United States, voodoo refers to the collection of spiritual practices developed in the South, primarily in Louisiana, that combines different rituals and spiritual beliefs of various practices, including Ifá, Kongo cosmology, Haitian Vodou, and Christianity. During enslavement, belief in voodoo was common among enslaved Africans. People who claimed to possess spiritual power through voodoo or hoodoo were considered to be the most powerful people on the plantation. Voodoo involved a deep understanding of the power of plants. It was common for people to use voodoo as a means to both heal and harm.[21]

The ability to heal and harm earned practitioners the title of "two-headed doctor." Often referred to as rootworkers or conjurers, they were revered for their knowledge about the physical and spiritual manifestations of illness. Practicing rootwork along with spiritual beliefs based in Kongo cosmology is known as hoodoo.

Enslaved Africans associated both hoodoo and voodoo with tricking, poisoning, and other forms of magical manipulation.[22] The power and mystery of the hoodoo was both feared and revered. After emancipation, belief in hoodoo and voodoo increased. Black people felt the freedom to practice their spiritual beliefs out in the open without fear of being watched by their masters.[23] Black people formed their own unique religious communities that incorporated Christian beliefs with Black spiritual traditions.

THE BLACK CHURCH

Religion and spirituality have always been a means to cultivate community. Outside of ATRs and ADRs, Christianity became a community-building tool for Black Americans. In a 1971 conversation with Nikki Giovanni, James Baldwin discusses the ways Black people, and Black Americans specifically, reimagined Christianity and the church in their own image. When talking about the power of "The Black Church," Baldwin says to Giovanni, "Baby, what we did with Jesus was not supposed to happen,"[24] specifically referencing the way Black American Christianity incorporates Afro-Indigenous ways of worship into the structure of the religion.

I grew up in a deeply religious family. My mom's side has been Baptist for as long as they can remember. When my parents started dating, my dad changed denominations from his family's Pentecostal beliefs to Baptist. In their youth, both my parents attended church regularly and were active members in their church community. Both my grandmother Louise and my grandmother Sandra attended church service almost every Sunday while my grandfathers stayed home.

I don't have very many clear memories of going to church as a child. My brother and I were active children with demanding schedules. Our weekends were often filled with ballet classes, soccer games, volleyball tournaments, and track meets. The more involved we were in extracurricular activities, the less we attended church—except on Easter. A few weeks before Easter, my mom would pick me and my brother up from school and drive straight to the mall. Hours passed as my mom riffled through the girls formal dress section at JCPenney, Macy's, and Robinsons-May, pulling out pastel-colored dresses made of layers and layers of tulle. As a kid, I dreaded the uncomfortable dresses, the endless photos, and the hours of church service. Despite never believing in the Easter bunny, I was still excited to see the elaborate Easter baskets my mom put together every year, decorate Easter eggs, and compete against my cousin during our family's backyard Easter egg hunt. I'd sit through church services, reminding myself of all the candy and fun that awaited me as soon as it finished.

Wherever I attended church, I felt deeply uncomfortable, like an outsider. I never understood how people found comfort in religion. From the ominous iconography to the concept of eternal hellfire, everything about Christianity made my hair stand on end. Church also turned my parents into scarier and more serious versions of themselves. Embarrassed to always be the new people in the congregation—they'd shop around for different churches each time they entered a new churchgoing phase—my parents took their frustrations out on my brother and me. Anything my brother and I did that might draw unnecessary attention to our family was scrutinized. My dad would angrily side-eye us if we were unable to sing along to songs that my brother and I never had a chance to learn. My mom, on the other hand, ignored us most of the service. It felt as if she were trying to mentally distance herself from us to prevent us from embarrassing her by association.

Our sporadic attendance also meant that my brother and I often felt overwhelmed by the culture of the Black Church. Watching elderly women "catch the Holy Ghost" terrified me. I never felt any euphoric religious experiences, and I was never swept up by the gospel music. I couldn't understand where the intense euphoria was coming from, I just knew that I didn't want it to happen to me. Too afraid to embarrass myself or my parents, I never felt free enough to get into the musical culture at church. It was only at home, when my mom played gospel music on our old black boombox while she made breakfast on the weekends, did I feel free enough to fully feel the power and beauty of gospel music.

Even though church was never for me, I grew to appreciate the culture of the Black Church the older I got. Around my junior year of high school, my parents, still testing out different churches, decided to attend a predominantly white Protestant church. Most of the kids I went to school with were Catholic, so my only concept of non-Black church was through stories I heard from them about attending mass. I'm not sure what I expected a non-Black Protestant church service to be like, but I was certainly shocked at what I experienced. I always felt that attending Black churches with my family was boring and tedious because the service seemed to drag on forever. Even though the white Protestant church service was shorter, I was bored beyond belief. Without the music and dancing and the pastor's lively sermons, I struggled through the hour and half service. Nothing about that experience felt recognizable to the churches I had previously attended. It felt so different it was almost like experiencing two different religions, and in many ways I was.

The Black Church is a term that evolved from the term *The Negro Church,* originally coined by W. E. B. Du Bois in his sociological study of the same title. In his report, Du Bois explores the origins of the Black Church, tracing its roots to indigenous West African spiritual practices.[25] He used the term *The Negro Church* to describe historically Black Protestant institutions, all of varying denominations but with similar cultural traditions. The seven major Black denominations are the National Baptist Convention, the

National Baptist Convention of America, the Progressive National Convention, the African Methodist Episcopal Church, the African Methodist Episcopal Zion Church, the Christian Methodist Episcopal Church, and the Church of God in Christ. At the time his report was published, Black American Christians didn't identify with each other or "the Negro Church," instead identifying by denomination.[26]

It can be said that enslaved Africans molded Christianity to fit their purposes more than Christianity molded them. Though Christian missionaries attempted to convert colonized and enslaved Africans, "conversion rarely entails the complete abandonment of former belief systems."[27] As in Kongo, enslaved Africans in the Americas interpreted Christianity through their own pre-existing worldviews. The Christianity of Black people across the diaspora is not the same Christianity of the white Protestants that converted them.

What makes the Black Church so unique is its incorporation of African spiritual practices in both covert and obvious ways. Through the lens of West and Central African spiritual practices, Black people's experience with Christianity involves a more tangible connection to spiritual power. In ATRs and ADRs, devotees are able to interact directly with spiritual forces through spiritual possession, known as "mounting." In Yoruba, priests that have been mounted are referred to as *esin orisa*, "the horse of the orisa."[28] Spiritual possession is referred to as "mounting" because it mimics the process of mounting a horse. In Ifá cosmology, spiritual possession occurs when the orisa's *emi*, animating spirit or "the breath of life," temporarily displaces the emi of the devotee. Any behavior performed from that point forward, until it is clear that the devotee's emi has returned, is assumed to be the actions of the orisa. After witnessing the Haitian lwa Guedé "mounting" devotees, Zora Neale Hurston recounts the first words spoken by the possessed: "'Parlay Cheval Ou' (Tell My Horse), the loa begins to dictate through the lips of his mount."[29] To be mounted is to invite the orisa or lwa to take temporary possession of the practitioner's body, usually through the interplay of drumming, ritual, and ecstatic dance. Drumming is an important component of mounting because it creates a trancelike atmosphere among participants in the ceremony.

Spiritual release is manifested through ecstatic dance. Choreographed dances that honor the orisa are different from the dances of possessed devotees. Once mounted, the orisa moves through the devotee's body in large forceful movements. In Yoruba, the word *kikan* is sometimes used to describe the forceful percussive nature of the dance. *Kikan* is an idiophonic word; the "up" tonality of *ki* and the "down" tonality of *kan* are used as onomatopoeia to describe the up and down movements that mounted devotees perform.[30]

Mounting is an important component of ATRs and ADRs because it provides an opportunity for the community to speak directly with the orisa, lwa, or spirit that is possessing the body of the devotee. During a mounting, the possessing spirit can speak through the devotee, communicating information from the spiritual world.

When the orisa leaves the inner head of the devotee, attendants rush to their side to help them as they come to. To help the devotee return to themselves, attendants will pour or spray their head with gin and reposition the devotee's body while calling their name repeatedly until they respond. Once recovered, the devotee often takes several minutes to sit and collect themselves before getting up and rejoining the group.

All the core elements of spiritual mounting are replicated in "catching" the Holy Ghost or the Holy Spirit in Black churches. Similarly to the use of the word *mount, catch* describes the way the worshipers interact with the Holy Ghost. In this context, catching is not synonymous with possession. It describes the overwhelming feelings of joy and ecstasy worshippers feel when they are in the presence of the Christian god. When worshippers catch the Holy Ghost, they begin to dance erratically. The energy in the room feels almost contagious, as more and more people begin to get swept up by the music. It's common for multiple people to catch the Holy Ghost at the same time, whipping the entire congregation into what W. E. B. Du Bois described as a "frenzy."[31] Attendants fan and cradle the worshippers who've caught the Holy Ghost until they've calmed down. Everything from the dance movements to the percussive music to the behavior of the congregation mirrors ritual possession in traditions like Ifá and Vodou.

The Black Church's early formation can be traced back to the praise house. Developed during enslavement, the praise house was the spiritual epicenter of Black plantation life. Praise houses were usually modest constructions built by plantation owners as a means of social control. By constructing praise houses within the plantation property, plantation owners attempted to prevent enslaved people from gathering with other enslaved people from neighboring plantations. Within the praise house, the ring shout, a type of dance and song ritual practiced by enslaved Africans in the United States and the Caribbean, was performed.[32] Blending various West African traditions from the Yoruba, Kongo, and Fon, the ring shout is often regarded as an example of Black spiritual resistance. Practitioners of the ring shout sing and dance while moving in a counterclockwise circle. The lead of the song would sing out a verse and everyone else would sing the response.[33] Call-and-response praise and worship is a key part of Ifá. Both Isese and Lukumi songs are sung in a call-and-response pattern. The leader, often but not always the babalawo or iyanifa, will sing a few verses of the song. The other practitioners will then repeat back some of the same lines sung by whoever is leading the song. Within Black churches, this tradition can be found in both praise songs and the way the audience relates to the preacher. The preacher will often orate in a song-like manner, and the audience will respond with affirmations. This back-and-forth dialogue between the spiritual leader is a unique component of African forms of worship.

The praise house's location and construction afforded enslaved Africans the liberty of movement. Hidden in the woods, the praise house gave enslaved Africans a place to worship away from the watchful eyes of white enslavers.[34] The praise house was the beginning of the Black Church's legacy as the epicenter of Black resistance in America. Enslaved Africans plotted rebellions and planned escapes from plantations within the praise house walls. The Black Church's role in Black resistance continued throughout history, playing a major role in the civil rights movement, birthing organizations like the Southern Christian Leadership Conference and leaders like Martin Luther King Jr.

WEALTH AS COMMUNITY

Wealth, in the way it is conceptualized within Ifá, has the ability to fundamentally shape communities on a relational basis. When we focus on building communal wealth, we are able to pour our efforts into cultivating deep and meaningful relationships that have the power to transform and are the basis of movement building. Through mutual aid, radical relationships, and organizing, we're able to work together to imagine new futures while supporting each other.

Community organizing creates a revolutionary sense of joy that Nick Montgomery and carla bergman call "joyful militancy," the emergent willingness to fight and defend that grows from an atmosphere that enhances the creative capabilities of those involved in struggle. Joyful militancy is rooted in anarchistic ideals of self-determination and experimentation. Joyful militancy is an inherently creative process, not rooted in fixed ideals of right or wrong.[35] It requires organizers to remain flexible and adaptable, not married to a particular ideology or tactic. The fluidity and flexibility inherent in the philosophy of ATRs and ADRs encourage practitioners to remain open-minded and receptive to different tools and techniques. Adopting that philosophy into community organizing strengthens organizers' ability to build coalitions with community members from diverse backgrounds and perspectives.

One of the greatest examples of joyful militancy is community organizing efforts during the civil rights movement. The Student Nonviolent Coordinating Committee (SNCC), Southern Christian Leadership Conference (SCLC), and the Congress of Racial Equality (CORE) were three of the leading racial justice organizations during the civil rights movement. Made up of a large contingent of university students from metropolitan cities, these organizations pioneered the use of nonviolence as an organizing tactic.

As part of their strategizing to increase voter registration in Southern states, SNCC, SCLC, and CORE sent student organizers to live with families in rural communities to build coalitions on the ground. Coming from major cities, many of these student organizers were unfamiliar with the reality of living in the Jim Crow South. Self-defense, not nonviolence, was the local strategy of Black residents. The violent threats from local police, the KKK, and angry white residents necessitated a strategy of self-defense. The very presence of student organizers fighting to increase voter registration and to end desegregation intensified the threat of white retaliation, putting the entire community at risk. In his book *This Nonviolent Stuff'll Get You Killed*, Charles E. Cobb Jr. illustrates various examples that highlight the magnitude of white violence on Black communities, often resulting in shootouts, bombings, police brutality, and KKK-led mobs. Faced with these new realities, both the student organizers and the rural Southern households they lived in had to determine which tactic would provide them with the best chances of survival.

The beauty of civil rights organizing was the ability to form coalitions between nonviolent student organizers and local residents, and the deep bonds formed were not only crucial to the success of the movement but also demonstrated the need for flexibility in terms of their tactics and ideology. Cobb describes a Black liberation movement marked by a foundation of community, trust, and common goals, not by ideology. Many of the young student organizers had their own ideology rooted in nonviolence, and while Southern residents respected the students' desire for nonviolence, they taught them the importance of self-defense in the cultural climate of the South. In *This Nonviolent Stuff'll Get You Killed*, student organizer Amzie Moses described his experience as a student organizer in the rural South: "Everywhere we went I and other civil rights workers were adopted and nurtured, even protected as though we were family. We were the community's children, and that closeness rendered moot the label of 'outside agitator.'"[36] Organizers in the Deep South recalled moments when the families that housed them used violent means to ensure their protection. Although many of the organizers themselves didn't carry guns, Black residents in the community disregarded these stipulations and opinions, opting to defend "the community's children." Had they come to the South attempting to change the local traditions of the community they sought to struggle alongside, their goals of increased voter registration and desegregation would not have been successful, especially in white supremacist strongholds throughout the South.

Civil rights workers had virtually no chance of successfully challenging local traditions of keeping guns for protection. Indeed, the issue did not even come up for most organizers, because the work itself—primarily organizing within the black community in rural areas—made the question of nonviolence moot. The ordinary day-to-day interactions of community organizing consisted mainly of attempting to persuade people to try to register to vote, and the question of nonviolence almost never came up.[37]

The ever-changing decisions and tactics employed by various Black organizers and leaders when faced with violence exemplifies the power of joyful militancy. At its core, anarchy is about experimentation; it's about reimagining new ways of living that are situationally determined, and not a prescribed set of notions for all to follow. Too often, white anarchist movements limit their imaginative capabilities by focusing too heavily on ideological frameworks and positions. Cobb reminds us that Black anarchism is ever-changing and adaptable. There is no one or right way of reaching a particular goal, but a multitude of strategies, tactics, practices, and beliefs that come together at different moments in time and history to propel the movement forward toward a common goal of liberation.

FOOD CULTURE ACROSS THE DIASPORA

My family always gathered around food. Any excuse to come together meant cooking a big meal. My extended family celebrated most holidays, but the main food holidays were the Fourth of July, Thanksgiving, Christmas, and New Year's Day. The Fourth of July called for barbecue. My dad or my uncle would grill up an assortment of meats, seafood, and veggies while my mom and grandmother prepared potato salad and corn on the cob. While my family cooked, I played in the backyard with my brother and cousins.

I helped out with cooking during the holidays. Growing up, my mom hosted Thanksgiving while both my grandmothers hosted Christmas. On Thanksgiving, my mom did the majority of the cooking, with some help from my grandmother Louise, my aunt, and me. The kitchen became a stressful place during the holidays, and I didn't always enjoy cooking. I was always worried that I was going to mess up a recipe in a catastrophic way. Usually, my grandmother would assign me to hors d'oeuvres, which were impossible to mess up. She skewered cubed cheese, ham, and olives to little toothpicks that she laid out on a plate. Hours before guests arrived, I would sit at the table carefully assembling each hors d'oeuvre. Aside from the turkey and ham, the women in my family cooked collard greens, black-eyed peas, candied yams with mini marshmallows on top, stuffing, and mac and cheese. Duck was my grandfather's and my favorite. Since my mom didn't cook duck most years, it felt like an extra special occasion when it was on the menu. In addition to sweet potato pie, which was my aunt's signature dish, other desserts my family made included cheesecake, bread pudding, German chocolate cake, shortbread cookies, and 7-Up cake. My mom typically made her famous Oreo cheesecake and German chocolate cake, while my grandmother prepared the 7-Up cake.

Christmas was my favorite time of the year. On Christmas Day, my parents split our time between my grandmother Louise's house and my grandmother Sandra's house. Christmas at my grandmother Louise's meant elaborate decorations inside and outside the house. Every year my grandfather climbed onto the roof to install Christmas lights in the form of the massive star of Bethlehem. My grandmother would wrap the trees in her front yard in tin foil and thick red velvet ribbon, turning them into giant candy canes. Christmas dinner consisted of most of the same foods we had at Thanksgiving with a few additions like mashed potatoes and crescent rolls. I made sure to save room for more food when we arrived at my grandmother Sandra's house. Every year, my grandmother would make deviled crab baked in little foil cups. I could easily eat a dozen deviled crabs in one sitting. My grandmother liked to eat her collard greens with hot sauce or with a little banana pepper. I likely developed a love for spicy food from adding banana peppers to my greens like my grandmother.

New Year's Day was a casual holiday for my family, usually spent with my immediate family and my grandparents. On New Year's Eve, my mom spent the day cleaning and tidying up the house so she wouldn't "sweep away" all her blessings in the New Year. On New Year's Day, my mom cooked corn bread, collard greens, and black-eyed peas to usher in prosperity in the new year. According to my grandmother Louise, corn bread represents gold, collard greens represent cash, and black-eyed peas represent coins. Eating black-eyed peas and collard greens is a common New Year's tradition in African American households that connects us to hoodoo traditions developed during enslavement.[38] Practitioners of hoodoo see the power in plants and animals, creating herbal remedies and recipes with spiritual intention. The lasting power of our food traditions is further evidence of our deep connection to the spiritual cultures that shaped Black life across the diaspora.

Outside the holidays, my family dinners consisted of spaghetti (a Black household staple), jambalaya, marinated chicken, and summer seafood boils. Jambalaya remains one of my favorite dishes. My family added seasoned chicken, sausage, and shrimp to a pan of rice that was cooked in chicken broth and mixed in onions, bell peppers, stewed tomatoes, and spices to bring it all together. My mom and grandmother fried fish often, typically catfish or trout. My favorite was fried trout, which my grandmother prepared by descaling and fileting a trout, coating it in cornmeal and spices, and frying it in a pan. I always saved the crispy trout skin for last because it was my favorite part. Every Halloween, just as the weather started to cool down, my mom would make a large pot of chili with corn bread for my brother and me before we went out to trick-or-treat. Winters called for beef stews packed with wholesome veggies and rich flavor. Less frequently, my mom would make other Southern staples like hush puppies, étouffée, and gumbo.

Most of the dishes my family prepares use a combination of African, European, and American ingredients and techniques. West Africans brought a deep understanding of plants, animal husbandry, and food preparation with them during the transatlantic slave trade. Animal sacrifice is a common practice in Ifá and other West African spiritual traditions. Before animals are sacrificed, prayers are recited to honor the spirit of the animal and to ask the orisa to accept the offering. After animals are sacrificed, they're cooked and eaten by the community. All parts of the animal are used and skillfully prepared. Black diasporans retained this knowledge of animal husbandry and food preparation, incorporating different animal parts into the dishes they made. My grandmother cooked oxtails, neck bone, chitlins (pig intestines), and pig ears for my mom and her siblings growing up. Utilizing all parts of the animal is a common practice among different indigenous communities. During enslavement, enslavers saved the best cuts of meat for themselves while the less desirable parts of the animal were given to enslaved Africans. Drawing from a rich culinary history, spiritual traditions of animal sacrifice, and indigenous food practices, enslaved Africans created dishes that combined ingredients from around the world while retaining a uniquely African flavor.

On their property, my grandparents and their relatives in Alabama raised chickens, pigs, and cows, animals that have a long history in African and African diasporan diets. Archaeological evidence suggests that guinea fowl particularly were domesticated two thousand years ago in what is now Mali and Sudan. In West Africa, guinea fowl is served with root vegetables like cassava, with rice, or with various stews. In the United States, poultry became a major part of enslaved Africans' diets. Fearful that enslaved Africans would buy their freedom with profits made from selling animals, the 1692 Virginia General Assembly outlawed the ownership of horses, cattle, or pigs for enslaved Africans. Chickens, however, were not mentioned.[39] At George Washington's Mount Vernon, enslaved Africans were forbidden from raising ducks or geese, making chicken the only type of poultry available to them. Over time, Black Americans, both enslaved and free, developed a reputation as chicken merchants.[40] Combining West African culinary practices, Black Americans fried, stewed, and marinated chicken, developing dishes like fried chicken and chicken liver with onions. In Jamaica, the blend of African and Taíno culinary techniques led to the creation of jerk chicken. Jerk refers to both the seasoning technique and the blend of spices used to prepare meat. Black people fleeing slavery formed maroon communities in the Jamaican mountains, creating settlements with the Indigenous communities that lived there. Traditionally used for pork, jerk preparation was eventually used for chicken and other meats.[41]

Pigs have a long history in Haiti, playing a central role in Haitian spirituality, food, and autonomy. Haitian farmers bred the Creole pig, suited for the particularities of Haiti's climate. Nearly 85 percent of rural households

in Haiti raised pigs, making it a central component of the Haitian economy.[42] In 1791 a Vodou ceremony held at Bois Caïman involved the sacrifice of a pig, marking the beginning of the Haitian Revolution. After an
outbreak of African swine flu, the US government, along with the Canadian
and Mexican governments, launched a program to eradicate Creole pigs.
Known as PEPPADEP, the program launched in the 1980s to curtail the
spread of African swine flu in the Dominican Republic from reaching the
United States and neighboring nations.[43] Over 400,000 Creole pigs were
culled over a thirteen-month period. The governments responsible for
PEPPADEP promised to replace Creole pigs with "better" pigs from Iowa.
The imported pigs were more expensive to care for, making them an unten-
able option for rural farmers. The year after imported pigs were introduced,
school enrollment rates dropped by 30 to 50 percent because rural families could no longer afford the cost of tuition and uniforms.[44] Pork is still a
major part of Haitian cuisine. One of Haiti's most popular dishes is griot, a
pork-based dish prepared by marinating pork in a mixture of orange juice
and lime, cooking it until tender, then frying it and serving it with a salad.[45]

Okra, groundnuts, black-eyed peas, cassava, plantain, yams, kola nuts,
millet, sorghum, cotton, watermelon, hibiscus, palm oil, Guinea grass, African eggplant, coffee, tamarind, and Akee apples are among the major crops
transported from Africa to the Caribbean and the Americas during the
transatlantic slave trade. Rice and cotton became cash crops in the American south, particularly in South Carolina, which profited not only from
the trade in enslaved Africans but also from African crops. Throughout the
Americas, especially Latin America, where the climate was similar to that
of West and Central Africa, African crops became foundational to Southern
American and Latin American cuisine.

Creole food is the African-influenced cuisine of Louisiana and the Sea
Islands off the Carolina Coast, both areas that historically served as ports
for trafficked Africans and previously the territory of British, Spanish, and
French colonial rule, which means the cuisine of these regions are heavily
influenced by African, Spanish, French, and Haitian flavors and are very
rich in seafood. These regions are known for retaining the most African
culture among Black Americans due to the geographical isolation of the Sea

Islands. The Gullah people are known for having a rich linguistic, spiritual, and cultural tradition heavily influenced by Igbo culture of Nigeria and Barbados,[46] while Louisiana creole culture relies heavily on West African and Haitian influences.

Drawing heavily from West African crops (okra, rice, black-eyed peas, and others) and West African food preparation techniques (stews, fried, mashed), Creole cuisine incorporated French flavors (roux, mirepoix, baguettes) to make one of the best culinary cultures in the United States. Gumbo, one of the most popular Creole-Gullah dishes, gets its name from the French word for okra, *gombo*. The English word *okra* comes from its Igbo name, *okuru*.[47] In West Africa, okra is used in soups and stews as a thickening agent. Popular creole dishes include shrimp and grits, oyster po'boys, jambalaya, oyster grits, deviled crab, crawfish étouffée, peanut cake, stews, and monkey bread.

Fufu, thought to have originated in Ghana, is a West African food made by pounding starchy tubers, typically cassava, yam, or plantain, with hot water to make a thick mashed paste. Known as *eba* in Nigeria, fufu is eaten across West Africa in places like Cameroon, Togo, Benin, and Sierra Leone.[48] Fufu is typically eaten with stews or saucy dishes like okra soup, tomato stew, or *egusi*. Fufu variants have made their way to Latin America and the Caribbean via the transatlantic slave trade. In the Dominican Republic, *mangú* is made by mashing plantains with butter or oil then boiled in water and topped with red onion and commonly served with breakfast. In Puerto Rico, mofongo is made by mashing plantains with garlic and topping it with chicharron, shrimp or other seafood, or chicken. In Mexico, *mogo mogo* (also called *machuco*) is a sweet plantain puree from the Tuxtla region of Veracruz. Machuco is also a popular Honduran dish of a slightly different variation.

In Ifá and Lukumi, certain foods are prepared as offerings for the orisa. Each orisa has preferred food offerings and taboos associated with certain foods. Obatala, for example, enjoys snails and coconut but never palm wine. Esu prefers offerings of palm oil, while Ọṣun and Yemayá prefer melons like pumpkin and watermelon. In Brazil, black-eyed pea fritters are both a popular street food and offering for the *orixas* Exu, Xango, and Iansa (Esu,

Shango or Chango, and Ọya in Ifá and Lukumi). Candomblé devotees pre-pare fried fish for Iemanja (Yemayá or Yemọja).[49] In Ifá, the Odu Ika Meji speaks about the power of the yam. Yams are sacred symbols for longev-ity because of their regenerative capability and their ability to grow easily throughout the West African climate.

CONCLUSION

The history of Black people is marked by migration. Our origins can be traced back to the birth of humanity, beginning somewhere in East Africa. From there we migrated throughout the continent, and eventually around the world. Across the African continent we built civilizations both commu-nal and hierarchical. The spiritual traditions we created were rooted in a reverence for nature, ancestors, and community. Our ancestors were fish-erfolk, artists, and farmers that shaped the West African economy, from small-scale communities to empires.

The transatlantic slave trade disrupted our ways of life, leading to the forced migration and enslavement of millions of West and West-Central Africans to the Americas. Our economies were destroyed in the name of "god, glory, and gold," fueling the economic advancement of Europe and the Americas. Our captors attempted to eradicate our indigenous beliefs and destroy our histories. To subjugate us, they stripped us of our humanity, transforming us into a people with no mother and no homeland.

We were reborn in the Atlantic, transformed into a new group of people born from struggle and cultural diversity. Our ancestors braided, swal-lowed, and smuggled seeds into their bodies, carrying the cultural, spir-itual, and culinary histories of West Africa to the New World. Ancestors like Adechina and many unnamed others fought to preserve our spiritual traditions. From Yoruba, Fon, Kongo, and Akan influence we reimagined Indigenous traditions in the Americas. Through improvisation and tech-nique, we created culinary and spiritual "jazz," blending together different approaches to food preparation and spiritual science. We fed our orisas and we fed ourselves with the seeds we planted in new soil. Gumbo, black-eyed pea fritters, and grilled pork are as much a part of us as hoodoo, Candomblé, and Vodou.

Capitalism and Christianity worked in tandem to colonize the African continent, transporting us on slave ships bearing Christian names. Decolonization requires us to interrogate the role of Christianity in the enslavement of African people and the continued role Christianity plays in our community. Labeling our ancestors as demonic aids in the mission of colonization, convincing us to willingly disconnect from our ancestral traditions. The majority of our ancestors had indigenous practices that were demonized and disregarded by the church. Even in Black churches, the impact of Afro-Indigenous practices can be felt in the ways Black Christians worship. Through spiritual possession and call and response, we can trace the roots of the Black Church back to the shores of Africa.

Our indigenous traditions combined with our history as the human capital and currency of the West remind us that true wealth is not achieved through colonization and capitalism. Wealth is rooted in the rich cultures and communities that sustain us and generate lasting legacies. If we continue to aspire to Western and capitalistic markers of success, we will continue to replicate the same systems of violence that have oppressed us for generations.

At its core the concept of Àjé is about abundance. Within ourselves, we have the skills and knowledge to create a world free from the violence and theft that created the world we currently live in. Our history is overflowing with examples of resistance and autonomy, from the religions we created to the animals we raised. The forced migration that created the diaspora taught us how to build communities and coalitions with diverse groups of people. Taking lessons from the civil rights movement, we can learn how to build community coalitions that are based on a shared common goal rather than an ideology. As we chart a path toward liberation, we can't fall into the traps of trying to replicate what was done before. We can incorporate lessons from our ancestors and study the strategies they used to survive, but ultimately it is up to us to create a new path forward. We have to remain adaptable and flexible for whatever future challenges come our way and remind ourselves of the joy that comes from community care.

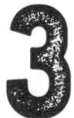

3

THE BLESSING OF ỌKỌ/AYA

You say I'm a woman and colored. Ain't that the same as being a man?
—TONI MORRISON, *SULA*

The idea of "body" carries this weapon: gender circumscribes the body, "protects" it from becoming limitless, from claiming the infinite vast, from realizing its true potential.
—LEGACY RUSSELL, *GLITCH FEMINISM: A MANIFESTO*

Family serves as the core organizing unit within cultures around the world. It represents the first collective of people coming together based on shared interests, common goals, proximity, and affection. From there, families form communities that then give birth to tribes and nation-states. For this reason, the family is often at the center of political arguments. We're frequently inundated with news stories and claims from conservative media that the family is in danger from one modern threat or another, usually sparked by the political organizing work of women, queer communities, and BIPOC communities. Much of this conversation revolves around the idea that the nuclear family as we know it will not be able to withstand political shifts in favor of women's rights, queer and trans rights, and racial justice.

In Ifá the family is supposed to be able to withstand outside forces, political shifts, and changing interpersonal dynamics. As described earlier, blessings in Ifá follow a system similar to a hierarchy of needs. Ire Ọkọ (the blessing of a husband) and Ire Aya (the blessing of a wife) set the foundation for the family and precede Ire Ọmọ (the blessing of children). When you combine the terms together, Ire Ọkọ and Ire Aya become the blessing of companionship or the blessing of partnership. As I will discuss in the following chapter, children are seen as communal wealth, a symbol of longevity, and the manifestation of victory. To unlock the blessing of children, one must first unlock the blessing of partnership.

A central concept in Ifá is the idea of being in alignment with one's destiny. Practitioners are constantly seeking guidance on how to remain in alignment with their destiny. Everyone's destiny is tied to their orí and is selected in Orun (the spiritual realm) before they are reincarnated into Aye (the physical realm or earth). Partnership is therefore seen as a divinely informed decision that should result in people choosing partners that help them on their journey to fulfill their life's destiny. A modern reframing of this concept focuses on choosing a partner that encourages you to grow, supports you in your goals, and is aligned with you mentally, emotionally, and spiritually so that you can continue to grow together.

I prefer to discuss Ire Ọkọ/Ire Aya in terms of blessings of partnership rather than blessings of a husband or wife for several reasons. The terms *husband* and *wife* are not only highly gendered but also place a premium on relationships that result in marriage. The Western concepts of husband and wife don't fit neatly into a precolonial Yoruba concept of partnership, nor does the modern concept of marriage. African and African diasporic communities have consistently practiced nontraditional ways of partnership and familial organization that are rooted in a cultural understanding of gender and family that depart from the West. As a queer person, it's important to me that I continue to investigate alternative modes of being related to gender and partnership through the lens of Ifá.

I've always had a complicated relationship with gender. As a young child, I didn't give my gender much thought. I was more concerned with self-differentiation, focusing my energy on forming an identity rooted in hobbies and early childhood interests. I found my identity in many activities that were deemed "girlish." I loved fashion, had an extensive Barbie doll and Bratz doll collection, and spent my days making potions from leaves and twigs I harvested in my backyard. I spent my early childhood forming close relationships with my boy cousins, one two grades above me and the other two grades below. Being so close in age, we did everything together. Our parents enrolled us in the same swim classes and soccer clubs, took us to watch the same movies, and bought us the same toys for Christmas.

Our only point of contrast was the way they dressed us. Even from a young age I felt like my mom wanted a daughter so she would have someone to play dress-up with. She often recounted stories of playing with paper dolls as a young girl, and I often felt that I was merely a paper doll personified. Every chance she got, my mom dressed me in pinks and purples; adorned my hair in barrettes, beads, and balls; and took me to the nail salon for manicures and pedicures. While I enjoyed the luxuriousness of the nail and hair salons, I despised the restriction barrettes and light-colored clothing imposed on my ability to freely experiment with the limits of my body. I spent my time on the playground playing house, doing cartwheels and roundoffs, and racing and wrestling boys. I often came home from school or my cousins' house with grass-stained knees and missing hair accessories, much to my mother's dismay. In one of my earliest memories of grappling with my gender expression and identity, I was in third grade, standing in the girls bathroom, looking into the mirror with a friend, and telling her that I was a tomboy. She looked at me in the mirror, giggled, and said, "There's no way you're a tomboy, dressed like that." I remember feeling upset and a little irritated by her comment. I didn't realize how much my outward appearance informed what people thought about me, regardless of my personality or my internal concept of self.

GENDER AS A SOCIAL CONSTRUCT

You've probably heard the phrase "gender is a social construct" used to describe the ways in which gender is not a fixed aspect of biology but an ever-changing and evolving form of performance and expression based largely on the contextual environment. The best definition of gender I've come across is from Oyèrónké Oyěwùmí in their book *The Invention of Women: Making an African Sense of Western Gender Discourses.* In this book, Oyèrónké dives into the Yoruba concept of gender by examining the Yoruba language. Oyèrónké states that

> gender is not a property of an individual or a body in and of itself by itself. . . . Gender is best understood as an institution that establishes patterns of expectations for individuals [based on their body-type], orders the social processes of everyday life, and is built into the major social organizations of society, such as the economy, ideology, the family, and politics.[1]

What Oyèrónké speaks to with this quote is the way that gender is entirely context-dependent, which allows it to change across generations, geographies, languages, races, and economic classes. In each of these varying contexts, gender looks a little different. When I would teach diversity, equity, and inclusion workshops, I helped people better understand the contextual nature of gender by posing a simple thought experiment. I would ask people to think about a young woman in England in the 1300s. I would invite them to imagine what she was wearing, how she spent her time, and what her life may have looked like. I then invited people to imagine a young woman in the United States in the present day. How might that woman's clothing, hobbies, and life differ from the English woman in the 1300s? All of the major markers of gender (clothing, interests and hobbies, social sphere) would look drastically different from one time period to the next. When a widely held social concept or belief is subject to change based on the context, that's typically a good indicator that that concept is socially constructed.

Oxford Dictionary defines a social construct as "a concept or perception of something based on the collective views developed and maintained within a society or social group; a social phenomenon or convention originating within and cultivated by society or a particular social group, as opposed to existing inherently or naturally." To say that a particular concept is socially constructed is to simply say that that concept is maintained by shared social beliefs rather than a material reality. A lot of political and cultural debate tends to focus on social constructs that are related to human characteristics. Usually, the divide lies between two frames of thought. The constructionist view argues that the basis for categorizing human characteristics is produced by culture rather than something biologically or naturally produced. This view acknowledges the contextual nature of gender and other human characteristics like race, criminality, and class and the role the geopolitical environment plays in shaping the way we talk about human characteristics. Biological determinists argue the opposite, positing that human traits are determined by the physical or genetic manifestation of the body. Biological determinists believe that the differences between people in terms of race and gender, for example, are rooted in a biological reality that results in distinct physical, psychological, emotional, and behavioral differences between different groups of people. Different cultures tend to lean more constructionist or more biological determinist based on their prevailing concept of social categories like gender, the family, and property, which is often reflected in language.

Biological Determinism

In the Western world, social identities are inherited and enshrined in the body. Biological determinism, the idea that your physical body controls and determines human behavior, is the primary basis for building social constructs in the West, where your body determines your social positioning; criminality, educational attainment, employment or lack thereof, marriage, offices held and positions of power are all perceived to be determined by the physical appearance of the body. Phrenology, hip-to-waist ratio, and BMI are "scientific" examples of how enshrined biological determinism is in Western society. Western philosophical culture centers around the idea that the visual is reality, popularized by the phrase "seeing is believing." The physical body provides visual "proof" of who an individual is, what they are capable of, and who they might become.

This hyper-focus on the body can be seen by studying European languages. Language shapes our worldview and our worldview shapes our language. The use of gendered pronouns in European languages specifically informs the lens through which speakers see and experience the world. Gendered pronouns (he/she, él/ella, elle/il) and gendered nouns (*la table* versus *le bateau, la flor* versus *el coche*) emphasize the gender binary in inescapable ways. This feeds into the idea of the universality of gender or gendered distinctions. From a Western perspective, all men and women, regardless of culture, have similar desires, and therefore similar struggles. Western nonintersectional feminist discourse attempts to universally apply "gender politics" to regions, cultures, and bodies where gender isn't conceptualized in the same way. Countless times, well-meaning white feminists from the United States have either ignored the nuanced struggles of Black women and women of color or have overgeneralized their own struggles, assuming that they apply to everyone. Examples of this include the struggle for women to enter the workplace, which focused on white, upper-class, and upwardly mobile women's realities, ignoring or overlooking the realities of Black women, women of color, immigrant women, and low-income women who were already full participants in the workplace.

Londa Schiebinger explores the Western preoccupation with the body as it applies to race and gender in her book *Nature's Body: Gender in the Making of Modern Science.* Londa paints a picture of the early biological sciences and the absurd, and sometimes funny, lengths European men went to "prove" their worldview through scientific study. Londa argues that "science is a product of society"[2] and that what we know and understand about the world is influenced by our cultural, political, and religious values. In the early European concept of "natural law," the precursor to the biological sciences, a clear distinction was made between natural law and the positive law of nations. Natural law was seen as an immutable fact, ordained by god. Humans', specifically men's, role was merely to uncover god's mysteries through the study of science. There are countless stories of early scientists using both implicit and explicit human sexual metaphors to describe plant anatomy and reproduction. When early botanist Carl Linnaeus developed the Linnaean system of classification, which groups plants into classes, orders, and genera, he based it on the physical differences between the male and female parts of flowers.[3] While it can be said that Linnaeus was one of the first European scientists to recognize the biological importance of sexual reproduction in plants, his system of classification focused specifically on reproductive organs rather than fundamental sexual functions. His system also baked in male hierarchy. The number of stamens (male reproductive organs in flowers) determined the class of the plant, while the number of pistils (female reproductive organs in flowers) determined the order. In Linnaean classification, class is placed above order. Linnaeus's decision to give male reproductive parts priority in determining the classification of an organism had no scientific justification.[4] He simply saw nature through the lens of the social relations that governed Europe at the time.

Linnaeus continued to draw from his understanding of social relations by personifying sexual reproduction in plants. As he began introducing new terms into his classification system, he added to the names of his classes and orders the suffixes -andria and -gynia, derived from the Greek words aner (husband) and gyne (wife). In his journals he describes plant sexual reproduction as an embrace between wedded couples. He writes, "The flowers' leaves . . . serve as bridal beds which the Creator has so gloriously arranged, adorned with such noble bed curtains, and perfumed with so many soft scents that the bridegroom with his bride might there celebrate their nuptials with so much the greater solemnity."[5] Along with many other early botanists and biologists, Linnaeus heavily used metaphor throughout the research. Many of these metaphors involved romantic interactions between plants or animals. Linnaeus continued with the metaphor of marriage by classifying plants as either monogamous (monandria) or polygamous (polygamia), depending on the arrangement of the pistils and stamens of the flower.[6] These examples illustrate the ways the social-cultural environment of Europe bled into early scientific understandings of biology, reproduction, and gender.

In the late seventeenth and early eighteenth centuries, botany and anatomy were taught in universities as two branches of medicine. This era of the scientific revolution was focused on finding universal laws of nature that could sum up all the variation in the world into a few neat concepts. Early scientists relied on analogies between plants, animals, society, and religion as they attempted to uncover these universal laws. During this period, the older Galenic "one-sex" model, which viewed women as a less perfect version of men, gave way to the "two-sex" model, which saw men and women as two distinct groups. Early anatomists sought evidence of sexual dimorphism, which was epitomized by illustrations of distinctly female skeletons in the mid-1700s.[7] The body became the proof of differences between the sexes, and these differences informed and were informed by the ways men and women were expected to behave in European society.

YORUBA AND GENDER

When I began studying Ifá and the Yoruba language, I was struck by how much gender neutrality came up as a recurring theme throughout the tradition and language. Language is a social institution shaped by culture. To better understand a culture, it's important to understand the way language embeds cultural values. In the second chapter of *The Invention of Women*, Oyèrónké explores the way Yoruba society was organized compared to the West. Prior to colonization, gender was not an organizing principle.[8] Rather than use gendered distinctions to organize society, the Yoruba, along with many other West African ethnic groups, had age-based societies. Seniority and relative age were used to confer status to individuals. Oyèrónké argues that the lack of gendered pronouns in the Yoruba language lends evidence to the claim that gender was not the main organizing principle in the precolonial era. In Yoruba, most names and all pronouns are gender-neutral. The pronouns *ó* and *wọ́n* are best described as informal and formal versions of the gender-neutral *they* in English. These are the only third-person pronouns in Yoruba. Similarly to the formal and informal *you* in French and Spanish, *wọ́n* is used as a sign of respect for older people or for someone with more seniority, whereas *ó* is used casually.[9]

Based on the lack of gendered pronouns in Yoruba, Oyèrónké argues that translating *obìnrin* to "female" or "woman" and *ọkùnrin* to "male" or "man" are mistranslations that ignore the etymology of Yoruba words in an attempt to find quick and easy English counterparts. There are no words in the English language that accurately capture the essence of the meaning of *obìnrin* and *ọkùnrin*. The common suffix *-rin* suggests a common humanity, whereas the prefix *obin-* and *okun-* speak to differences in anatomy and reproductive function.[10] The Yoruba concept ọkùnrin, which refers to "maleness" in anatomical and reproductive function, is not seen as the norm or as representative of humanity as a whole; conversely, in English, we use the word *man* to describe both male or masculine people as well as humanity in its entirety. *Man* in the English context is seen as the default, and everything that falls outside that category is an outlier. In Yoruba, the word *ènìyàn* is the nongendered word for humans. The use of the word *ènìyàn* places both obìnrin and ọkùnrin on the same level conceptually. Ọkùnrin is not seen as more privileged than obìnrin, while *man* and *maleness* in English are considered to be at the highest rank. Obìnrin doesn't correspond to connotations of subordination and powerlessness in relation to ọkùnrin.

Oyèrónké also points out that unlike English and other European languages, Yoruba only applies reproductive distinctions to adults. There's no gendered word to differentiate between children in Yoruba. In English we use the words *boy* and *girl* to distinguish between male or masculine and female or feminine children. In Yoruba, the word ọmọ is used to describe a child of any gender. Siblings are distinguished by relative age rather than gender. Classifiers like *àbúrò* and *ègbón* are used to distinguish between younger and older siblings, respectively.

Gendered words are also not applied to *eranko* (animals) or *ewé* (plants) in Yoruba. The terms *akọ* and *abo* are used to describe differences between animals, plants, and abstract periods in time. Though *akọ* and *abo* refer to "fruitlessness" and "fruitfulness," respectively, they are not posited as opposites. For example, an *akọ ìbépẹ* is a papaya tree that does not bear fruit, but it would be incorrect to call a papaya tree that does bear fruit an *abo ìbépẹ*. Bearing fruit is considered the norm for papaya trees, so a fruitful papaya tree would just be considered an *ìbépẹ*. When speaking about a fruitful or productive year, someone might use the phrase "*odún t'ó ya 'bo*." The phrase "May your year be fruitful" (*ya 'bo*) is commonly used to wish people a happy new year. Yoruba New Year falls in June and coincides with the arrival of new yams, emphasizing the correlation between fruitfulness and positive outcomes for the year.[11] It would be incorrect, however, to refer to a bad year with the term *akọ*.

The way abo and akọ are not opposites or compliments in Yoruba reflects the way that obìnrin and ọkùnrin are also not conceptualized as opposites or compliments. The best way to describe obìnrin and ọkùnrin in English is to define *obìnrin* as "anatomic female" and *ọkùnrin* as "anatomic male." Unlike the English words *male* and *female*, obìnrin and ọkùnrin don't hold any real cultural meaning beyond reproduction and are not associated with gender stereotypes related to physical, mental, emotional, or spiritual differences. Oyèrónkẹ́ argues that the terms *obìnrin* and *ọkùnrin* speak purely to the apparent physical differences between the two anatomies. They don't express sexual dimorphism or gender categories and speak only to reproduction.

What Yoruba society and language demonstrate is an alternative world that relies on social relations rather than the body. Yoruba society reminds us that it's possible to acknowledge differences in anatomy and reproductive role without using those differences to codify social ranking. Biology is limited to reproductive matters but holds little to no weight outside of that realm.

Taking a look at Yoruba cosmology, orí, the spiritual "head" that exists within everyone and is selected in Orun before an individual reincarnates onto Aye (earth), has no gender. When selecting one's orí, the focus is on choosing an orí that has a good fate or an orí that will lead you to learn important lessons that will ultimately allow you and your lineage to continue to move closer to your destiny or higher purpose. The concept of choosing an orí is never concerned with gender or physical appearance.

In a Yoruba myth, there is a story of three friends who go to the divine potter Àjàlá to select their heads before their journey to earth. The gender of these individuals is irrelevant to the story. Two of the friends make hasty, superficial decisions leading them to select damaged orís that lead them to face struggle and loss on earth. The third friend takes their time inspecting the clay heads made by Àjàlá, and through their patience and thoroughness, chooses a well-made and fully formed orí that allows them to prosper on earth.[12] The lesson of this odu is meant to highlight the importance of the orí-inú (inner head) in shaping one's fate and destiny. The orí is a central concept in Ifá. Shrines are built for practitioners to worship their own orí and are used by practitioners to ask their orí-inú for guidance. These shrines are highly decorated, typically with beads and cowrie shells, and look the same regardless of the gender of the person it belongs to. The concept of a genderless inner divinity that lives within each of us differs from traditional Western concepts of gender. In the West, gender is both a physical and internal manifestation of oneself. In precolonial Yoruba society, there is no inherent inner difference between people. The difference lies in the spiritual structure of one's orí and is not connected to anatomical or physical differences.

Yoruba is not the only gender-neutral language in West Africa. Many indigenous West African languages follow a similar gender-neutral structure, including Igbo, Wolof, and Akan. In *Male Daughters, Female Husbands: Gender and Sex in an African Society*, Ifi Amadiume argues that the gender neutrality found in the Igbo language represents the precolonial cultural understanding of gender. In Igbo, *oke* refers to an anatomic male and *nyi* refers to an anatomic female. Like Yoruba, Igbo uses the gender neutral pronoun *o* to describe both anatomic males and females. The word *mmadu*, meaning humanity, is applied to all people. In Igbo, the words *onye be, nwunye,* and *nwanyi* translate to "wife" but are also used to describe someone who doesn't own the home or someone who is in service to another.[13] These examples illustrate concepts of gender across West Africa that diverge from Western gender norms.

ORISAS AND GENDERQUEERNESS

When I began studying Ifá during 2020, I was initially intrigued by the presence of feminine orisas. A large part of my disillusionment with Christianity was the concept of a male god as the supreme ruler of the universe and the giver of life as we know it. Finding a tradition that worshiped Black feminine divinities was incredibly affirming. I lit a yellow Ọṣun votive candle often and spent hours scrolling on Pinterest for artistic depictions of Ọṣun, Ọya, and Yemayá. Never before had I found a tradition where I could see myself clearly reflected in the divine.

Ọṣun is often the first feminine orisa people are introduced to. Beyoncé's 2016 embodiment of Ọṣun during her music video for her song "Hold Up," where she's seen wearing a yellow dress and walking barefoot through water, remains one of the most popular recent representations of the Yoruba goddess. Like many other cultures with feminine deities, the mythology surrounding feminine Yoruba orisa doesn't align with traditional Western gender expectations and stereotypes. Ọṣun is known as the "mother of sweet waters" and is often associated throughout the diaspora with the divine feminine and concepts like love, romance, and beauty. However, in Isese Ifá, Ọṣun is not associated with love, beauty, or sexuality.

Ifá as a tradition is centered around the concept of longevity. Love, beauty, romance, and sexuality are all important yet fleeting aspects of human life. Orisas are not associated with fleeting concepts, especially if those concepts are not rooted in the natural world. Based on the odus, Ọṣun is the orisa of freshwater and is known for her ability to heal through the combined power of water and herbs. When you break down the word *Ọṣun*, the suffix -*ṣun* means "to ooze," "to seep out," or "to gradually flow from." The literal translation of Ọṣun is "the one who oozes [water]" or "the one from whom [water] oozes or springs from."[14] Ọṣun is specifically associated with fresh flowing rivers, with a major river in Nigeria named after her. The Ọṣun-Osogbo Sacred Grove is the site of a yearly pilgrimage where Ifá practitioners travel to honor the orisa. The grove is home to a large river and is regarded as one of the most sacred sites in Nigeria. Ọṣun serves as a reminder not to allow your own energy to become stagnant, and to embody coolness in terms of your character.

Though Ọṣun's reputation as a healer is probably the best-known aspect of her identity, Ọṣun is also known as both a diviner and a fighter. One of her sacred tools is a machete, allowing her to strike down her enemies as well as clear paths to usher in new energy and to lead to new avenues for growth. Her personification as a fighter defies traditional Western concepts about femininity, and her role as a diviner solidifies the intelligence and importance of women in Yoruba cosmology. Ọṣun's association with water and reflective materials (mirrors and brass) symbolizes balance. Ọṣun represents the balance of masculine and feminine energy, which she embodies

as a wife, mother, and *irunmole*. An irunmole is one of the primordial celes-
tial energies that were present during the formation of the earth. Ọṣun was
among the first irunmole and was the only feminine irunmole in existence.
In the Yoruba creation myth, the masculine irunmole were unsuccessful in
creating life on earth until they included Ọṣun. Her crucial role in creation
solidified Ọṣun as the source of all life. As the source of creation, Ọṣun's
role as a mother is referenced in various stories. As a mother, Ọṣun acts
as a portal, birthing all the potential possibilities of life into the physical
realm. Motherhood requires the balance of masculine and feminine energy,
since mothers are capable of creating all gender potentialities. As wife to
Ọ̀rúnmìlà, the orisa of divination, Ọṣun's healing energy provides balance
to Ọ̀rúnmìlà's wisdom. Together, the power of divination and healing work
together to outsmart the forces of iku (death).

Unlike Ọṣun, Ọya not only defies Western concepts about femininity,
she exists outside the bounds of gender. Ọya is a popular yet misunder-
stood orisa. In many songs throughout the diaspora, Ọya is referred to as
ayaba in reference to her relationship with Ṣàngó. *Ayaba* is a contraction
of the words *aya* (wife) and *oba* (ruler), translating to "wife of the ruler."
According to Yoruba mythology, Ṣàngó is a deified ruler of Oyo, an ancient
kingdom in what is now Nigeria. Together, Ṣàngó and Ọya form the counterparts of powerful forces that usher in change and victory. Ọya is associated with storms, the marketplace, and graveyards across the diaspora,
each symbolizing the powerful and disruptive forces of sudden change,
wealth, and death-rebirth. Similarly to Ọṣun, Ọya carries a machete, which
she uses to achieve victory during battle. Her association with change is
represented in stories that speak about her ability to shapeshift, changing
into different animals and morphing her gender. Known as a fierce warrior,
Ọya is said to grow a beard during battle to fight with the men.[15] Ọya's gen-
derplay enables her to embody the transitive nature of change and imper-
manence, illustrating the shifting boundaries of gender. To Ọya, gender
is a tool to be used in different circumstances, not a fixed state of being.
By performing masculinity by growing a beard, Ọya becomes powerful
enough to go to battle. The performance of gender is precisely what gives
gender power.

As I learned more about the tradition as well as other West African traditions, I was shocked to discover that "the creator" was often described as genderless. In Ifá, Olódùmarè is not a separate entity that exists outside of humanity and the cosmos. Olódùmarè is everything. The collection of all the beings, all the orisa, all the planets and stars that make up the universe is Olódùmarè. If the creator encompasses everything there is, then how could the creator have a gender? That would be like saying reality itself is masculine or feminine. Reality just is. Olódùmarè just is. This concept of a genderless creator unlocked something in me. If the truest nature of existence was genderless, then what did that mean for someone like me?

Similarly to Ọṣun, Olódùmarè represents all the potential possibilities in the universe. In the Yoruba context, creation and creative forces are genderless or represent a balance between masculine and feminine energies. Obatala, the orisa of creation, is often considered to be gender-fluid or genderless. Obatala consists of two words, *oba* (ruler, the one who presides over) and *tala* (white, undyed cloth). Obatala's mythology is a combination of the deification of one of the early rulers of Ife (an ancient kingdom in Nigeria) and the orisa Obatala. Obatala has many paths, or aspects, some feminine and some masculine. As the orisa responsible for molding the human form and due to his role in creating the earth, Obatala's gender fluidity is representative of his ability to create life.

THE CONCEPT OF "WIFE"

When I was in undergrad, the political landscape shifted. I found myself in the Obama-Trump era of identity politics and DEI workshops where, for better or for worse, identity was a core topic of conversation. Gender discourse and sex positivity were the focus of the campus events I attended and the books I read. In the process of working out my own feelings around gender and sexuality, I entered a series of tumultuous and short-lived sexual relationships. In these relationships, I found a sense of freedom. College was my first opportunity to explore my sexuality and gender identity. In dating men and women, I connected to a part of my identity that I had suppressed during my childhood. It felt liberating. By the end of college I was out to most of the important people in my life.

At the tail end of undergrad I met my partner. We began dating seriously around the time I started graduate school. Being in a relationship brought up a lot of complicated feelings about how I saw myself. I spent college casually dating, enjoying the freedom it gave me not to be tied down in a committed relationship. My relationship with my partner was the first time I could call someone my "boyfriend." It was a thrilling experience that often made it difficult for me to locate my emotional feelings about my relationship. I was clouded by the excitement of simply being in a relationship. Dating a cis-het man made me slowly slip into gendered patterns of interacting. I became increasingly consumed by the idea of being a "good girlfriend." I wanted to be feminine, sweet, charming. I stopped interrogating my gender identity and only spoke about my sexuality in a way that was alluring to my partner. It was cool to be bisexual now, and I felt that it gave me an edge and a sex appeal in the eyes of my partner. As our relationship solidified and life caught up to me, I stopped having the energy to keep up the ultrafeminine performance. I simultaneously felt more comfortable and more awkward than I ever had before. After years of ignoring the internal questions I had about my gender identity, I felt lost. I was unable to locate myself in the feminine gender performance I had taken on during my relationship. I began drifting back to the tomboyish energy of my youth, but this time I began expressing it through my clothes. I still felt feminine in many ways, but I was beginning to understand more clearly what people meant by the spectrum of gender identity.

As my concept of gender and partnership continued to evolve, I searched for a deeper meaning of the Yoruba concept of Ire Ọkọ/Ire Aya. The way my ilé speaks about the third blessing in Ifá is through the framing of the traditional nuclear family. Ire Ọkọ/Ire Aya are described as "the blessing of a husband/the blessing of a wife" and is seen as a precursor for the fourth blessing, Ire Ọmọ, the blessing of children. As a queer person with complicated feelings about both marriage and child-rearing, I was initially put off by the idea that a core tenet of Ifá involved striving toward ideals I was uncertain about. Studying ATRs specifically and indigenous religions generally is a complicated journey, especially for queer people new to these traditions. Colonization and influences from Christianity and Islam color much of the cultural landscape of West Africa and the diaspora. It's impossible to practice an ATR without encountering colonial or Abrahamic influences.

As Oyèrónké explains, many of the "gendered" words in Yoruba are mistranslations or misunderstandings of the complexity of Yoruba culture. For example, the words *iya* and *baba,* which translate to "mother" and "father," are less concerned with gender and more concerned with the concept of parenthood. In precolonial Yoruba society, the concept of parenthood was closely intertwined with adulthood. Similarly to the use of *wọn* to denote seniority and *obìnrin* and *ọkùnrin* to denote reproductive role, *iya* and *baba* are used for adults of reproductive age as well as parents. *Iya* and *baba* are categories of both adulthood and parenthood and are not constructed within a gender binary.

A similar case can be made for the terms *ọkọ and aya,* which loosely translate to "husband" and "wife," respectively. To grasp the full meaning of these words, it's important to understand the structure of precolonial Yoruba families and the concept of property. The *agbo ilé* was the primary social unit, essentially the housing compound that consists of members of a family who all claim to be descendants from the ancestor who "founded" the compound. These compounds extended beyond the Western nuclear family and included siblings, parents, wives, and children, creating a small community of relatives. Often these families specialized in a particular trade, such as smithing, dyeing, or weaving, and worked together to manage the family resources. All members of the lineage were collectively referred to as *ọmọ ilé* (children of the house) and were ranked by birth order. Marriage residence was determined patrilocally, meaning obìnrin would relocate to the family compound of the ọkùnrin they married. Obìnrin that married into the family were referred to as *aya ilé* and were ranked by marriage order. *Aya* was the term used to denote outsiders or nonowners who married into the family. The ọmọ ilé of the family were positioned as ọkọ in relation to the in-marrying aya, regardless of sex.[16] Mothers often referred to their children as *ọkọ 'mì* ("my ọkọ") as a term of endearment. This phrase signified their children's place in the family lineage in relation to their own. In Ifá, after being initiated into the house of a particular orisa, all devotees are referred to as aya of that orisa. The initiates are described as aya because they have "married into" the "house" of the orisa.[17] This indicates that ọkọ and *aya* are not inherently gendered terms but concepts associated with one's place within the family lineage.

Inheritance within the family lineage was ranked by both status and seniority. All ọkọ, regardless of sex, had priority over aya. When aya married into a family, they lost their age within that family and were essentially reset. They did, however, gain status in relation to other aya who married into the family after them. The constant reshuffling of seniority and marital status colored the interpersonal family dynamics of Yoruba life. Though it was common for aya to relocate to the family compound of the ọkọ, this relocation was not necessary or permanent. In some cases, obìnrin from noble families did not relocate to the ọkùnrin's family lineage. In some cases, an aya could return to their home of birth once child-rearing responsibilities were completed. There was no concept of a conjugal estate.[18] Each partner in the marriage was an ọkọ within their own family and stood to inherit their respective family's resources. Though there were general expectations for ọkọ and aya, the Yoruba concepts of marriage and family provide us with examples outside the Western perspective. These examples remind us that there exist limitless possibilities for how to structure society outside the gender binary.

GENDERQUEERNESS ACROSS THE DIASPORA

Learning about the inherent queerness and gender expansiveness of Ifá helped me come to terms with my gender and sexuality. Even though I felt like I had moved on from my childhood, I still had internalized homophobia and transphobia to work through. The environment of my childhood, tinged with racism, homophobia, and transphobia, left very little room for me to feel comfortable discovering and exploring my gender and sexuality. I found comfort in my relationship with my partner, both because it was loving and because it didn't challenge my internalized gender stereotypes. In my relationship, I fell into a compulsory heterosexual dynamic. I didn't have to interrogate the ways we were relating to each other. I could go into autopilot and follow the societal script laid out for me. I felt both a sense of protection and confinement in the heteronormative appearance of our relationship. For a while it worked, but over time the nagging thoughts I had drove me to confront my gender identity and the gender dynamics within our partnership. Together, my partner and I began approaching our relationship from a different perspective. We've made it a point to address the gender norms that show up in how we relate to each other and interrogate whether they still serve us.

What I sought was a "queering" of the prescribed gender dynamics that impacted my romantic partnership and my personal relationship to gender and sexuality. To be queer is a political act rooted in the rebellion against normative ways of relating in the aspects of life that are impacted by gender and sexuality. Although queerness is directly related to sexual and gender identity, it extends beyond that to encompass a political framework for relating. Queerness is a refusal of, or the inability to conform to, the prescribed status-quo. In the context of Eurocentric cultural narratives and the Western concept of gender, Blackness is "queered." Blackness serves as the barometer for what whiteness is not. Black and African ways of conceptualizing and performing gender diverge from Western gender ideals. These differences are what makes Blackness a "queered" identity in the West.

I found comfort in the gender fluidity of the orisas. The orisas serve as a reminder of other gender potentials and possibilities that exist outside the Western gender binary. They provide examples of "feminine" warriors, gender-fluid creators, and "masculine" mothers. As a child of Obatala, the owner of my head, I saw myself both in Obatala's creative energy and his gender diversity. Learning about gender neutral languages in West Africa reminded me that gender diversity is ancient. Our ancestors understood that gender exists on a spectrum. It's a flexible aspect of our inner selves, not something rooted in our bodies. As I continue my quest to better understand my ancestors, I'm deepening my understanding of myself.

THE IDEA OF WOMANHOOD

Narrow definitions of gender rooted in Western biological determinism pushed Black cis and trans women to the fringes of society. The construct of "womanhood" and "femininity" in the Western imagination does not have the space necessary to encompass the experiences of Black womanhood. As Saidiya Hartman states in *Wayward Lives, Beautiful Experiments*, "It was obvious that gender as category was not elastic enough to encompass the radical differences in the lived experience of black and white women."[19] The legacy of "slavery, stolen labor, violated flesh, and negated maternity" enshrined the differences between Black and white womanhood. The servitude, serial marriages, and spontaneous partnerships that defined Black women's lives in the twentieth century continued to widen the gap. In her book *Fearing the Black Body*, Sabrina Strings illustrates how religion and medicine worked in tandem to morph and change the ideal female body to always exclude Black women in one or more areas, namely hair, facial features, and bodyweight and shape. Strings argues that "since women have long been evaluated based largely on their physical appearance, racial-moral social distinctions primarily target the women in each racial/ethnic group."[20]

The greatest failure of Black women in the eyes of sociologists of the twentieth century was their status as breadwinners in their families and community. Black women acting as the breadwinners of their homes was seen as a threat to Black masculinity and a symptom of a dysfunctional family. Beginning in 1643, Black women's labor was classified the same as Black men's. The Virginia General Assembly taxed Black women's labor; taxation of labor was traditionally reserved for men in agricultural labor and the heads of households.[21] Since enslavement, Black women's labor has been treated the same as men's, marking Black women as deviant from traditional gender norms. Black women's role in the US workforce was born from enslavement and post-emancipation survival. The racialization of labor forced Black people into low-wage jobs, excluding them from the economic freedom white Protestant Americans experienced at the turn of the

century. A woman that didn't need a man raised questions about her societal status and gender.

Regardless of Black women's behavior, Western gender ideals necessitated the exclusion of Black women to bolster and uplift white womanhood
as the ideal. In an attempt to gain access to the status of "woman," some
Black women use hyperfemininity or transphobia in an attempt to distance themselves from women they deem as "less feminine." Whether Black
women "had bobbed hair or not, wore pants or dresses, had husbands or
not, it didn't seem to matter. . . . There was nothing the world wouldn't do
to a colored woman. Everything they did to Black men, they did to Black
women."[22] Race, gender, and sexuality form an interconnected web made up
of shifting rules and definitions that morph to fit the demands of the white
ruling class. The gender and sexual expression of Black and Indigenous
communities has been used as evidence to justify white supremacy. When
race and gender are conflated, it becomes clear that "the fidelity to gender
roles and the punishment of sexual variance [are] other ways of maintaining
and policing the color line."[23]

RITUAL GENDER PLAY

Gender play, which I define as the exploration of identity by assuming
hypergendered and hypersexed modes of interaction, is a central part of
African traditional and diasporic rituals. West African spiritual rituals often
involve elements of trance and spiritual possession. The transformative
power of ritual, meant to invoke the spirits and pierce through the veil that
divides the physical plane from the spiritual, provides a space for freedom
and play through dance and performance. Drums and highly percussive
instruments are expertly played to invoke trancelike states among ritual
participants. *Djembe, bata,* talking drums, and *udu* are all examples of different indigenous African drums used in various ritual performances. In Ifá,
specific orisa are associated with specific drums or specific drumming patterns. For example, Ọya is associated with *bembe* drumming, a specific type

of rhythmic pattern played on percussive instruments. A popular Yoruba song known throughout the diaspora speaks to Ọya's connection to drums:

> Bèmbé Ọya
> Ọya la fi ń dáa e
> Òrìrí
> Ọya, ìyá èwe (yewe)
> Ayaba

> Using Ọya's drums
> Ọya is who we often use to be good
> great, powerful, fierce wind
> Ọya, mother of children
> Wife of the leader (queen).[24]

This song illustrates the strong association between Ọya and bembe. Ọya's song is representative of the musical force behind ATR and ADR rituals. Chanting, singing, and drumming work together to invoke the orisa or lwa during ceremonies and performances. Once invoked, the orisa and the devotee are able to make contact, evidenced by ecstatic dance and elaborate gender performance.

Mounting, or spiritual possession, occurs when an orisa, lwa, or spirit enters the body of devotees during ritual dance. When an orisa or lwa takes possession of a devotee, they're recognized in the behavior and dances performed by the mounted devotee. Each orisa and lwa has signature behaviors and body language that identify them. Zora Neale Hurston describes the behaviors of Guedé, a Haitian lwa characterized by his sarcasm and overt sexual performances. Guedé, also referred to as Guedé Nibo, was formerly a human man who died a violent untimely death and was later deified. Guedé is known for wearing a black overcoat and hat, smoking cigars, and drinking rum infused with hot pepper and other herbs and spices. To identify a devotee who has been mounted by Guedé, the devotee is required to swallow some of the rum infused with hot pepper and then wash their face with it. According to Zora, "the faker will always draw back because he fears to get that raw rum and hot pepper in his eyes, while the subject really mounted will do it."[25]

Regardless of the gender of the devotee, the mounting spirit will manifest in similar ways through the devotee's behavior. Mounting transforms the devotee into the physical representation or conduit for the orisa. Mounted devotees are literally transformed into the gender of the possessing orisa. In *Yoruba Ritual: Performers, Play, Agency*, Margaret Thompson Drewal witnesses Iya Ṣàngó, a priestess of Ṣàngó who was initiated in the 1960s, during a ritual mounting. Through ritual, Iya Ṣàngó "literally becomes male . . . through possession trance." As Ṣàngó, Iya Ṣàngó plays with gender "enacting fucking with other men." This performance blurs the lines of the gender identity and sexuality of Orisa Ṣàngó, Iya Ṣàngó, and the audience. "Is she a woman constructing men as her objects as if she were male, or is she a man playing to other men as if they were women?"[26] Not only does the behavior of devotees change, so does their clothing. Drewal recalls the moment when a male practitioner gave a woman performing a masculine dance his clothing. When asked why, he replied that it was "to make the dance look fine."[27] Other examples of gender play include the use of prosthetic penises by women possessed by Esu. Male priests of Agemo, an orisa represented by the chameleon, wear their hair styled in traditionally feminine braids and enter the Agemo shrine dressed in feminine clothing. At its core, spiritual possession recognized the separation between the body and gender identity. Some aspect of the emi contains the essence of gender, since it is the emi that changes a devotee's behavior while in trance.

Ritual and ceremony provide a space where gender norms and expectations are shed. People are free to act and speak their minds, free of consequence. As Zora describes, being "under the whip and guidance of the spirit-rider" is a form of psychospiritual submission in which "the 'horse' does and says many things he or she would never have uttered un-ridden."[28] Spiritual possession provides a type of plausible deniability, where the possessed are not held accountable for their actions while under the influence of spirit, creating a space where people are free from any societal consequences that might otherwise arise from gender transgressions or divergence from any behavioral norms. Dance and possession within Black spiritual traditions serve as opportunities for freedom and release.

Gender in the Era of Enslavement

Gender was one of many tools enslaved Africans and free Black people used to evade detection, cross borders, and survive. In *Black on Both Sides,* C. Riley Snorton shifts through historical examples, describing the way "captive flesh [created] a critical genealogy for modern transness, as chattel persons gave rise to an understanding of gender as mutable and as an amendable form of being."[29] Enslaved Africans used gender as a tool for survival. There are several historical accounts of enslaved Africans dressing in ways that altered their gender appearance to evade capture. These include accounts describing "the different ways fugitives 'disguised in female attire' or 'dressed in the garb of men.'" One such example describes how Harriet Tubman disguised a Black man as a woman wearing a bonnet to help him escape arrest and reenslavement.[30]

Stories about "cross-dressing" captured the public's attention and quickly became a media sensation. An example is the story of Mary Jones, a Black sex worker living in New York in the 1800s. After Robert Haslem met with Mary Jones for a so-called "tour of pleasure," he realized his wallet was missing. With the help of another of Mary's clients, Haslem informed police, leading to Mary's arrest. Mary was tried for grand larceny in June 1836. Mary appeared in court in the women's clothes she was arrested in, prompting ridicule from the spectators. When asked in court about her clothing, Mary replied that she "always dressed in this way" and that it was the women who worked in the brothel that convinced her that she "looked so much better" in them. Mary makes a point to contextualize her appearance, stating that she "always attended parties among the people of [her] own Colour dressed in this way."[31] Mary was found guilty and sentenced to five years of hard labor. Following the trial, news of Mary's arrest spread through the media. Images of the "Man-Monster" began to circulate, depicting an average-looking Black woman with the caption "Peter Sewally alias Mary Jones &c &c." Newspapers speculated about the nature of her encounter with Robert Haslem, claiming that she wore a "'piece of cow [leather?] pierced and opened like a woman's womb . . . held up by a girdle,'" earning her the moniker "Beefsteak Pete."

In an attempt to reconcile with what Saidiya Hartman describes as the "violence of the archive,"[32] we can create speculative fiction of Mary's gender identity and make claims about the motivations behind her gender expression. Stories of enslaved and incarcerated Black people are often lost to history. The only records we have access to are the ones written by their enslavers and imprisoners. We are not able to definitively declare that Mary's gender performance is rooted in self-identification. What is evident is that "cross-dressing" created an experimental atmosphere between Mary and her clients by giving birth to emergent modes of relating.

The Turn of the Twentieth Century and the Harlem Renaissance

Hidden within the blurred gender roles that defined Black life at the turn of the twentieth century was a queer underground defined by the party culture at the center of urban life. Parties provided space for secretive and underground gatherings where Black queer community flourished. At the center of queer and countercultural nightlife was the cabaret. In an essay titled "The Cabaret as a Useful Social Institution," Chandler Owen describes the deeply human desire for food and sex, the latter of which can be partially satisfied through dance. Originating in France, the cabaret was the pinnacle of dance and performance in the late 1800s and early 1900s and served as a gathering place for dance, performance, and leftist ideals to proliferate. In the United States, jazz music was an influential component of cabaret nightlife. Jazz represented freedom, "unrestrained impulse," and "carnal desire."[33] The energy and excitement of jazz created a colorful nightlife that attracted a diverse and eclectic group of people. As Owen described it, the cabaret was one of the few institutions "breaking down the color line" and "destroying the psychology of caste."[34]

In this space of experimental music and experimental social norms, Black queer communities gathered. Between the cabaret, music halls, and private parties, "pansies, faggots, lady lovers, and bull daggers" found spaces to let loose and experiment in new ways of interacting and loving. Blues singers like Ma Rainey and Lucille Bogan sang explicitly queer lyrics, referencing rumors about their sexual orientation. In 1925 Ma Rainey was arrested on accusations of hosting a "lesbian party" in her home.[35] Rainey addressed the speculation about her sexual orientation in the song "Prove It on Me," singing

"I went out last night with a crowd of my friends / It must've been women, 'cause I don't like no men," daring listeners to prove the rumors about her to be true. Lucille Bogan's 1935 song "B.D. Woman's Blues" directly referenced her identity as a "bull dagger," Black slang for a butch lesbian. *Bull dagger* as a term alluded to a type of Black butch chivalry and sexual prowess. Bogan sings about the mistreatment bull daggers face from men, describing it as a "lowdown and dirty sin." She describes the gender expression of bull daggers evident in the way they walk and dance as being "just like a natural man."

The cabaret scene of the late 1800s bled into the Harlem Renaissance, which brought queer society to the larger popular culture. Marked by intellectual and social progress and experimentations, the Harlem Renaissance ushered in an era that celebrated Black cultural contributions. Writers like Langston Hughes, Zora Neale Hurston, and Countee Cullen were prominent figures of the Harlem Renaissance, publishing poetry, essays, and anthropological studies that highlighted the beauty and richness of Black life in America and throughout the diaspora. Rumors swirled as the public speculated about their sexuality. Though both Langston and Zora's sexual orientation was never confirmed, their failed marriages, close friendships with openly gay intellectuals like Alain LeRoy Locke, and intimate friendships that bordered on romantic relationships has earned them a place in Black queer history. Cabaret bars and clubs like Clam House hosted queer singers like Gladys Bentley, who wore a tuxedo and openly flirted with women.[36] Drag balls were hosted at places like the Savoy Ballroom. The drag balls of the early 1900s followed in the footsteps of parties hosted by William Dorsey Swann, the first queen of drag, who held secret masquerade balls in Washington, DC, in the 1880s. Swann's parties were frequently raided by the police, where they reported encountering Black men dressed in feminine attire.[37] The drag balls of the Harlem Renaissance were epicenters of partying and pageantry, with attendees dressing in elaborate outfits and participating in judged competitions.

From the Ballroom to Today

Ballroom culture continues in the centuries-long Black tradition of gender play through dance and performance. Harlem's reputation as an epicenter of queer culture would later give rise to the balls of the 1960s. Interracial drag pageants began in Harlem in the 1920s, with the most popular one hosted at Hamilton Lodge. The racism and colorism of the interracial drag pageants pushed Crystal LaBeija and Lottie LaBeija to host their own drag ball in the early 1970s. In the wake of the 1969 Stonewall riots, they hosted their first drag ball, called "Crystal & Lottie LaBeija Presents the First Annual House of LaBeija Ball." It marked the formation of the first drag ball "house," the House of LaBeija.[38] What followed was the birth of a uniquely Black and Latinx queer ball scene in New York. Others followed suit, forming their own houses, often named after major fashion brands. Houses act as both dance troupe and chosen family for queer youth whose biological families shunned them. As ballroom culture shifted from drag balls to house balls, houses competed against each other in categorized pageantry competitions and performances. In the late 1970s and early 1980s, ballroom legends Paris Dupree and Willi Ninja contributed to the creation of voguing, an improvisational dance inspired by the models' poses in popular fashion magazines. Over time, different styles of voguing evolved as new dance moves and techniques were incorporated.

There are three main styles of vogue dance: old way, which emulated poses from fashion magazines and Egyptian hieroglyphs; new way, which introduced elements of martial arts to old way vogue; and vogue fem, the post-1995 style of vogue characterized by traditionally feminine movements inspired by jazz, ballet, and modern dance.[39] Jennie Livingston's groundbreaking 1990 documentary *Paris Is Burning* illuminated the epicenter of ball culture, featuring famous ball legends like Willi Ninja, Paris Dupree, and Venus Xtravaganza. In recent years, drag and ballroom culture has reemerged in popular culture. Television's *RuPaul's Drag Race*, *Legendary*, and *Pose* are all examples of popular media that highlight the history and continuation of Black queer performance, music, and dance.

Black queer gatherings continue today in similar fashion to the parties of the nineteenth and twentieth centuries, bringing together an eclectic mix of fashion, dance, and spirituality. In Los Angeles, queer parties for Black and brown communities attract crowds of partygoers and popular music artists. Founded by Kumi James, known by their stage name BAE BAE, Hood Rave is an alternative Black dance party that centers Black queer and femme artists, DJs, and partygoers. BAE BAE describes Hood Rave as having an "energy on its own that's spiritual and [that] has the potential to be revolutionary."[40] BAE BAE co-runs Hood Rave with their close friend Kita Clark, known as DJ Kita, combining their knowledge of LA's underground music scene to curate an event by Black queer folks for Black queer folks. Raving has always been a spiritual experience, integrating dance music with countercultural movements. Hood Rave taps into the ancestral energy of Black ecstatic dance and queerness. Every part of Hood Rave is unapologetically Black, as BAE BAE and DJ Kita make it a point not to cater to the tastes of non-Black audiences. DJs and artists that perform at Hood Rave often remind partygoers that while the space is open to everyone, it's always Black femmes and queer folks to the front. BAE BAE describes the experience of being on the dance floor at Hood Rave as "really freeing." They speak about how the energy of the parties "feels ancestral—like we're tapping into something deeply rooted."[41] Hood Rave is one of many newer Black queer-centered parties and events popping up across the country. Like Hood Rave, these parties aim to create safer spaces for Black queer communities to gather.

HOMOPHOBIA IN AFRICA AND THE CARIBBEAN

While queer parties are flourishing in the United States, the safety of the LGBTQ+ community is threatened in many countries in the Caribbean and across the African continent. More than half of Africa's fifty-four countries prohibit same-sex activity. In the Caribbean, several countries have laws prohibiting buggery and gross indecency, aimed at prohibiting same-sex relations.[42] As of 2023, four countries, including Nigeria and Uganda, had laws that mandated that same-sex activity was punishable by a multiyear prison sentence and in some cases death.[43] Caribbean and African anti-LGBTQ+ laws and the cultural prevalence of homophobia and transphobia has made them among the most dangerous regions in the world for queer people.

Many of these laws can trace their roots to colonial influence from European nations. Of the seventeen African countries colonized by the

British, only three have ended their antigay laws. A 2014 study by the *Washington Post* revealed that former British colonies had a higher chance of having anti-LGBTQ+ laws. Researchers found that 70 percent of countries with British colonial origins continue to criminalize homosexuality.[44] Though colonization can account for many of the anti-LGBTQ+ laws, the recent wave of Western evangelical influence has resulted in increased criminalization of queer communities in various African nations. In the early 2000s, evangelical leaders of the US "ex-gay" movement, consisting of people who claim to be "reformed homosexuals" attempting to discourage people from engaging in same-sex relationships, flocked to Uganda to speak at several evangelical conferences. Scott Lively, a prominent evangelical from the United States and author of *The Pink Swastika: Homosexuality in the Nazi Party,* spoke with the Ugandan parliament, where he claimed that homosexuality was a Western import aimed at corrupting children. Using the same conservative talking points pushed by US politicians to justify anti-trans legislation, Lively, along with other evangelical leaders, successfully convinced Uganda's parliament of the supposed dangers of homosexuality, leading to Uganda's 2009 "Kill the gays" bill. This bill called for the death penalty for any acts deemed as "aggravated homosexuality."[45]

Though there are more spaces for Black queer communities to gather in the United States, violence against Black LGBTQ+ folks still persists. According to the Human Rights Campaign, 61 percent of murders of trans and genderqueer people in the United States were Black trans women. Texas and Florida, two states with some of the most extensive anti-LGBTQ+ laws, have the most reported fatalities of trans and genderqueer people, with thirty-seven murders reported in Texas and thirty-three in Florida since 2013. Despite California's anti-discrimination laws and policies, California ranks as the state with the third-highest number of fatalities, with twenty-five murders since 2013.[46] Violence against Black trans women occurs at the intersection of transphobia, homophobia, sexism, and patriarchal violence. Like African and Caribbean countries, colonization impacts the pervasiveness of homophobia and transphobia within Black American culture. The adoption of rigid gender norms rooted in Christian and colonial beliefs held within the Black American community fuels homophobic and transphobic violence.

Activists and organizers in the United States, the Caribbean, and Latin America continue to advocate for the safety and liberation of queer people throughout the diaspora. In Nigeria, activists raise money to provide gender-affirming clothing to queer communities through organizations like the Oasis Project. The Oasis Project connects queer Nigerians to mental health, housing, and medical support through their partnered service providers. In the United States, Black-trans led organization For the Gworls curates parties and raises funds to help Black trans people pay rent and pay for gender-affirming care. Brazilian dance collective Batekoo cultivates internationally recognized queer parties that seek to affirm LGBTQ+ Brazilians. Mixing Brazilian funk, hip-hop, and other music from the African diaspora, Batekoo has become a cultural phenomenon.[47] Through dance, Batekoo unapologetically reclaims space amid the homophobia and violence in Brazil.

CONCLUSION

Queer identities are shaped by the pursuit of freedom and beauty. Existing outside Western gender norms and societal expectations, Black queer people have created spaces for movement, expression, and play. We can locate ourselves in an ancestral understanding of gender that recognizes the dual humanity and divinity present in each of us. The gender-neutral languages of West Africa create a person-centered worldview that recognizes us all as ènìyàn. Men and women are seen as complements rather than opposites. When necessary, gender is one of the many tools we can use to evade capture, harking back to the myths about Ṣàngó and Ọya's gender transformations while also honoring the stories of enslaved Africans' pursuit of freedom.

We create new worlds of possibility, transforming ourselves through the improvisational dances of spiritual possession and voguing. Through queer parties I'm able to locate myself within the past traditions of my ancestors.

The familiar rhythm of house music awakens ancestral memories of the bembe.

If orisas of any gender can find homes within our bodies, we too can make space for the genderqueerness that lives within us. If Ifá is about honoring our orí and uplifting the divinity with us, unapologetic queerness is the embodied worship of our highest self. We can change and transform our bodies, clothes, and behaviors to make the dance of life "look fine" according to our own visions of self. In the pursuit of beauty and self-love, we dare to imagine alternative worlds by creating our own families, parties, and mutual aid networks.

If capitalism can be compared to gluttony and cannibalism, based in an insatiable desire that ultimately destroys the self, then queerness is a savoring of the self, indulging in a self-love that is regenerative rather than all-consuming.[48] Queerness is a radical act of self-love; we embrace the multitudes of Black identity.

Through the spiritual traditions of Ifá and Vodou, we're reminded that other ways of conceptualizing gender exist outside the West. We can incorporate lessons from the gender-neutral languages of West Africa as we imagine new ways and worlds free from homophobia and transphobia.

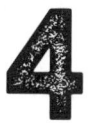

THE BLESSING OF ỌMỌ

We say that mothering, especially the mothering of children in oppressed groups, and especially the mothering to end war, to end capitalism, to end homophobia and to end patriarchy is a queer thing. . . . Those of us who nurture the lives of those children who are not supposed to exist, who are not supposed to grow up, who are revolutionary in their very beings are doing some of the most subversive work in the world. If we don't know it, the establishment does.

—ALEXIS PAULINE GUMBS, *REVOLUTIONARY MOTHERING: LOVE ON THE FRONT LINES*

My relationship to children and my political theory about child-rearing and how best to structure families come from my personal experiences within my own family, my experience working as a confidential youth advocate, and my doula training. Though I don't have children of my own, I'm deeply invested in the infrastructure and community we create for children. In Black cultures, children are considered to be the responsibility of the entire community. There are countless examples of neighbors, distant relatives, and "play cousins" creating a supportive community to raise Black children. I consider myself to be an integral part of that community.

My desire to see children thrive begins with my desire to see Black birthing people thrive. The reproductive justice movement is an integral part of advocating for rights for birthing people and children alike. Reproductive justice for Black women encompasses a wide range of topics, including the right to safe abortions, pre- and postnatal care that reduces maternal mortality rates, access to contraception and education about family planning, and safe and supportive communities to raise children free from violence and scrutiny.

Family lays the foundations for how children are raised and determines what people they will become when they interact with the world around them. The family is the institution from which all other institutions are born. Society is the sum of many families coming together. The rules and norms established within the family are designed to prepare children for survival in the outside world.[1] Black parents and caregivers struggle to prepare their children for a world that was not designed for them while simultaneously dealing with racism and other systemic forms of violence themselves. There's a delicate balance to be struck between providing Black children with tools to thrive in a white, capitalist world while grounding them in the beliefs and values central to self-determination and liberation. Most parents do the best they can with the limited tools they have. Each generation is faced with new hardships under the same system that strips us of our economic, emotional, and spiritual freedom.

My parents and grandparents worked hard to prepare my brother and me for dealing with all the ups and downs of life. Growing up in Los Angeles, my parents saw the ways gang violence and police brutality affected their communities. On January 23, 1990, my mom's childhood best friend Oliver Beasly was shot and killed by police in Los Angeles. Oliver was twenty-seven years old and was an active member in the Nation of Islam. His murder sparked outrage across the city, with thousands of people attending his funeral service.[2] Oliver's death has left a lasting impact on my mother. For my family, police violence wasn't something abstract. It directly influenced their lives and the lives of their community. I don't know all the reasons my parents had for leaving Los Angeles and moving to Orange County in the late 1990s. I know that they wanted better opportunities for my brother and me, and I'm sure that their personal stories colored their decision to leave.

When my parents moved us to Orange County, my aunt's family had just bought a home nearby, making it an ideal location for my parents to put down roots. I grew up surrounded by family. My cousin, aunts and uncles, and grandparents all lived in Southern California less than an hour's drive away. Most of my relatives moved away from Los Angeles to the suburbs in Orange County and the Inland Empire. My family chose suburbia for many of the same reasons as other families: better schools and cleaner neighborhoods. My parents thought little about the racial impact moving to a predominantly white neighborhood would have on my brother's and my upbringing.

To prepare us for the world, my parents emphasized the importance of education. School, piano, dance, and sports ruled my childhood. Though I enjoyed school and excelled academically, at times it felt like my academic achievements were the only thing my parents liked about me. I didn't always feel like I had the space to make mistakes and learn from my own experiences. My parents sheltered me from the outside world. To them, the world was dangerous and violent. It was best for me to stay home and focus on my studies. My parents' hopes and dreams were wrapped up in my successes and failures. I represented all of their hard work and effort, and I often felt pressured into molding myself to their tastes. My parents tried to provide me and my brother with opportunities and experiences they didn't have access to when they were growing. They used the tools and skills they had to the best of their abilities to prepare me and my brother for the world.

THE BLESSING OF CHILDREN

Following the blessing of Ire Ọkọ/Ire Aya is the blessing of Ire Ọmọ, the blessing of children. Ire Ọkọ/Ire Aya provide the foundation for Ire Ọmọ to manifest. Ọmọ and ọmọdé are the Yoruba words for child and children. While ọmọdé is typically used to describe young children, ọmọ is not age-specific and is used by parents or guardians to describe both young children and adult children. As mentioned in the previous chapter, there are no gendered words for children.

Ọmọ is broken down into two words: the prefix ọ-, which in this context means "the one that," and mọ, which means "builds," "molds," or "shapes." Ọmọ can be understood as both "the one who is molded" and as "the one who molds or shapes."[3] The meanings of the word ọmọ allude to the transformative nature of children and the transformative process of childhood. Children represent the future potential of a community and are seen as the manifestation of longevity, wealth, successful partnerships, and a prosperous community. As children learn and grow toward fulfilling their own destinies, they in turn shape the destiny of the world around them.

In Ifá, the idea of destiny is a driving force within the tradition. One's destiny is decided before incarnating on earth and is connected to one's orí, or highest self. A contract is formed between an individual's orí and Olódùmarè describing the individual's purpose and the lessons they intend to learn in their next life. Once a child is born, they forget their contract with Olódùmarè, and a divination ceremony called ẹsẹntaye is performed to mark the birth of the child and bring them into closer alignment with their destiny. During this ceremony, a child is given a name that is connected to the odu they receive through divination. If through divination it's determined that an orisa played a significant role in bringing the child from Orun (the ancestral or spiritual plane) to Aye (the physical realm), the orisa's name is incorporated into the name of the child. Names like Esubiyii and Ogunbiyii translate to "Esu gave birth to this one" and "Ògún gave birth to this one," respectively.[4] The odu given at birth holds spiritual significance and influence over the child's life and is connected to better understanding their destiny.[5] This odu will continue to be a strong guiding force for the path your life takes, unless you undergo various initiation ceremonies like receiving your Hand of Ifá or initiating to an orisa. Each initiation is a new rebirth, so any subsequent odus received during those ceremonies take precedence over the odu initially given at birth.

In Ifá cosmology, a newborn baby resides somewhere within the liminal space between Orun and Aye. The esentaiye ceremony, which provides clarity on how best to welcome the baby into the physical realm, often includes instructions for the parents on how best to raise their child, including taboos—things to be avoided to ensure optimal success in life.

They can range from warning parents against fighting around the baby to cautioning parents about what foods or activities to avoid during the first years of their baby's life. The taboos determined at divination serve as a mini manual for child-rearing for new parents, providing them with insight into how to conduct themselves and how to ensure the safety of their child. *Yoruba Ritual: Performers, Play, Agency* shows us an example of a diviner explaining to new parents that their baby's orí-inú (inner head) is closely connected to *ifi* reeds that grow near bodies of water. He warns the parents about bringing the baby close to water and instructs them not to let the baby sit on mats made of ifi reeds.[6]

Children are deeply connected to the concepts of àìkú (longevity) and rebirth. In Ifá, reincarnation typically occurs within a lineage. When an ancestor is recognized in a young child, they are sometimes given the names *babatunde* or *iyatunde*, meaning, "father has returned" or "mother has returned." This concept is explored in Akwaeke Emezi's novel *The Death of Vivek Oji.*[7] Vivek's grandmother passed away the same day as Vivek's birth. Their connection was visibly manifested in a birthmark on Vivek's foot that matched a scar Vivek's grandmother had in the same place. The theme of Vivek's grandmother returning in Vivek's body plays a central role in the character's exploration of their sexuality and gender identity throughout the novel.

Unlike other reincarnation-based spiritual practices like Buddhism, Ifá practitioners are not trying to escape reincarnation. Reincarnation is seen as part of the cycle of all things in the universe and is one manifestation of the balancing of universal forces of light and dark, death and rebirth. The goal is to continue the cycle of reincarnation as a way of continuing the ancestral lineage. Children are the embodiment of the spiritual evolution from the ancestral realm to the physical.

Though all children are seen as blessings in Ifá, twins hold special significance. Ibeji (also spelled Ibeyi) refers to the sacred twin orisa. Twins are a common symbol in West African cosmology, likely due to the high rate of twin births in West Africa. In Nigeria, 45 out of every 1,000 births is a twin birth compared to the global average of 12 out of 1,000.[8] Ibeji are closely associated with Ṣàngó, symbolizing double blessings, wealth, and victory. When twin babies are born, they're given the names Taiwo and Kehinde, corresponding to the age of the twin. *Taiwo* loosely translates to "the one that tastes the earth" and is the name given to the baby that is born first. *Kehinde* translates to "the one that comes last." Though Taiwo is the first born, in Yoruba cultural cosmology Taiwo is considered the younger twin. In Yoruba cosmology, as the oldest child, Kehinde sends Taiwo out of the womb first to see if everything is OK. Ibeji is typically represented as two twin statues, one an ǫkùnrin and the other an obìnrin, further emphasizing the concept of duality.

BIRTH WORK ACROSS THE DIASPORA

For as long as I can remember, I've been both fascinated and terrified by childbirth. As a biologist, I was always curious about conception and pregnancy. It was exciting and terrifying to learn about the ways a person's body changes when they're pregnant, how their organs move aside to make room for the life growing inside them. I wanted to learn more about the electrical and chemical reactions that happen during conception. On the other hand, I was terrified about the process of childbirth. In my undergraduate evolutionary endocrinology class, we spent half of the semester watching birthing videos from around the world. Different cultures, practices, and traditions highlighted the many different birthing techniques. This class sparked my interest in alternative birthing practices. I was interested in the ways indigenous women around the world gave birth. I was struck by how the birthing positions indigenous women used looked radically different from birthing positions in the United States. So much knowledge and wisdom was passed down from women, generation after generation, creating a sacred medical tradition.

My fear and fascination culminated with me beginning doula training in 2021. After working in nonprofits for a few years, I wanted to explore another avenue for working with communities that allowed me to provide a direct service without the limiting bureaucratic structures many nonprofits are forced to navigate. Doulas serve as support during significant transitional processes in life. Most commonly, doulas are thought of in the context of birth, but there are several different types of doulas, including abortion doulas, death doulas, and transition doulas, to name a few. Abortion doulas support people through the process of abortions, typically providing both emotional support and physical care. They often talk with clients in advance, accompany clients to the procedure, and assist with aftercare, such as preparing meals and ensuring they have a comfortable place to recover. Death doulas support people on their transition at the end of their lives. Many death doulas work with clients who have terminal illnesses, often meeting with them for a few months to several weeks before they pass to help emotionally prepare them for their end-of-life transition. Transition doulas provide support and care during the process of gender-affirming care, which typically involves medical interventions such as hormone therapy or gender-affirming surgery.

Doulas and midwives are often conflated, when in reality they are two separate and distinct roles. Unlike midwives, birth doulas do not aid in anything "below the waist" during birth. Birth doulas are responsible for providing emotional, physical, and informational support before, during, and shortly after birth.[9] Doulas are particularly helpful in terms of informational support and advocacy for new parents.

Doulas also provide support by informing the client of different birthing positions and the tools available in each setting. Through my classes, I learned more about different birthing practices and techniques from around the world. My teacher incorporated lessons from indigenous midwives and doulas. We learned that squatting was the primary birthing position used by indigenous people around the world. My instructor also introduced us to the use of the rebozo before, during, and after labor. A hand-woven shawl typically worn by Indigenous women in Mexico, the rebozo can be tied around the waist to support the belly and ease pressure during pregnancy. It can also be used during labor to help turn the baby to ensure it is positioned head-down. After birth, it can be tied intricately around the waist to help support the abdominal muscles. Doulas typically carry bags that include rebozos and other tools that can help support the client during labor.

Doulas are especially helpful for Black and Indigenous women in the United States. According to the Centers for Disease Control and Prevention, in the United States as of 2022 Black women are 2.6 times more likely to die in childbirth while Indigenous American women are twice as likely to die during childbirth as white women.[10] Although this is an improvement from 2021 Black maternal mortality rates, Black women continue to die at a higher rate than any other racial group in the country. Among several recommendations aimed at reducing Black and Indigenous maternal mortality rates, the CDC's "Hear Her" campaign is specifically targeted at improving the lines of communication between pregnant women and their health care providers. Increased medical interventions have been linked to birth complications such as cardiac arrest, blood clots, infections, and death, which are three times more likely to occur following a C-section. Women that are supported by doulas are less likely to require C-sections or use pain medication; they have shorter labor times and report higher birth experience satisfaction.[11]

More Black and Indigenous women are seeking the support of doulas and midwives to improve their overall experience and reduce the risks associated with childbirth in the United States. Currently, over 90 percent of practicing midwives are white, emphasizing the racial barriers Black people face when seeking medical care.[12] Prior to the twentieth century, the majority of midwives in the United States were Black. Traditionally, midwives were typically women that provided care to women during labor throughout Asia, Africa, Latin America, Europe, and North America. Prior to the Civil War, Black midwives made up half the midwife population, while white and Indigenous midwives made up the other half. These women worked alongside more experienced midwives, learning through an apprenticeship model. Enslaved Black women worked as midwives for both enslaved women and their enslavers. They sometimes were allowed to travel and receive payment. Beyond providing care during labor, Black midwives often served as full-spectrum health care providers for women, administering traditional herbal birth controls and abortifacients.

Part of the certification process requires an apprenticeship with a doula so that you can shadow them as part of your training. After searching for several weeks, I finally connected with Mandi, a Black full-spectrum doula who worked with a variety of clients in Santa Barbara, California, serving both wealthy families and low-income women. She works closely with doulas and midwives that speak Spanish to better serve the Latinx community. One of my first lessons focused on helping Mandi prepare a postpartum package for a client. I arrived at Mandi's house nervous yet eager to learn. Our task for the day was to cook placenta in preparation for it to be powdered and packaged into pills for the new mom. Over the course of several hours, we cleaned, cooked, and dehydrated the placenta. With the increased interest in alternative and traditional birthing practices in the United States, many birthing people are opting to consume their placentas after birth. While medical evidence is scarce, some people believe that eating the placenta provides the birthing person with nutrients that aid in the recovery after birth.

Holding the placenta in my hand, I was struck by the viscerality of birth. I had little experience with pregnancy and birth outside my coursework. Seeing a placenta close up transformed birth from a mysterious process into a real biological phenomenon. After washing it thoroughly in the sink, Mandi prepared a mix of fresh ginger and spices. We seasoned the placenta and placed it in a steamer to cook for about an hour. After it was cooked, we sliced it into strips and placed it on a vegetable dehydrator. Mandi told me that while this client preferred to consume her placenta in pill form, Mandi had worked with clients who preferred to have it incorporated into a meal. A few days later, after the placenta was fully dehydrated, Mandi ground up the strips in a coffee grinder specifically designated for processing placenta, and filled vegetable gel caps with the powder. She delivered the pills to the new mom to take over the course of several weeks. In some indigenous communities in Nigeria, the placenta is typically buried on the family compound or the compound of the attending midwife. There are a number of reasons why different cultures bury the placenta after birth, some spiritual and some practical. Most of the spiritual reasons are related to the connection that both the placenta and the land has to ancestors.

In Nigeria and among many indigenous cultures, traditional childbirth is a process led by women (obìnrin) specially trained in traditional midwifery. Though different tribes practiced different traditions surrounding birth, women in several different tribes typically underwent birthing rituals or gave birth on their mother's compound, which was typically the compound of their birth. Among the Igbo, women underwent a series of elaborate rituals that both ushered her into womanhood and motherhood. Performed by women in her mother's compound, the new bride and soon-to-be mother participated in the "tying the wrapper" ceremony that marked the transition to womanhood, symbolized by moving from just wearing traditional waist beads to wearing a wrapper that covered most of the body. She was then given a small painted doll to carry in a bag around her waist, symbolizing future children. Until at least her first child was born, the new bride carried the small doll with her at all times, receiving blessings and well-wishes from women everywhere she went.[13]

Unlike in the West, women don't lie on their backs during traditional births. Lying on your back with your legs up during the birthing process places the center of gravity at your lower back, making it particularly cumbersome to push the baby through the birth canal. The pelvis also becomes misaligned, causing the opening of the canal to become contracted. The traditional birthing position in Nigeria is to squat with the assistance of birth attendants.[14] Squatting aligns the pelvis and hips and places the center of gravity directly in alignment with the birth canal. This eases the birthing process by allowing the birthing person to push with, rather than against, gravity.

The traditional birthing position also holds spiritual significance in Ifá. When devotees greet orisa shrines, they often place their foreheads on the ground both to honor the orisa of the shrine and to honor Aye, the orisa that is the earth herself. When a baby is born in the squatting position, their head is the first part of their body to touch the earth. By touching their head to the earth, newborns are saluting and acknowledging Aye, honoring her for welcoming them to the physical realm. Other spiritually significant parts of birth involve the amniotic sac and the umbilical cord. In Ifá cosmology, white cloth is a recurring motif throughout the tradition. Connected to Obatala, the orisa of creativity who is said to have molded all humans in Orun, white cloth symbolizes the nobility and purity of the orisa. The white cloth worn by devotees and used during ritual ceremonies is also said to represent the birth caul, the amniotic sac that surrounds a baby in utero.[15]

Wearing white cloth is symbolic of both the many rebirths that initiates undergo in the tradition as well as the youthfulness of devotees in relation to the primordial spirits.

In extremely rare circumstances, babies are born "en caul," meaning that the amniotic sac is still intact with the baby when it is born. En caul births occur in 1 in 80,000 births and hold spiritual significance in many cultures.[16] During all other births, the amniotic sac breaks, signifying the moment the birthing person's water breaks. The breaking of the amniotic sac represents the first blessing a child receives from Ọṣun, the orisa of sweet waters, in the form of the sacred waters of the womb. En caul births are sometimes referred to as "veiled births." The veil refers to the thin divide between the physical and spiritual worlds. According to Yoruba tradition, babies born en caul are given the name Ọ̀kẹ́, which means "sack." These babies are considered to possess spiritual gifts because they are able to see beyond the veil. It's often predicted that babies born en caul will grow into great spiritual leaders or become leaders of some significance in their communities.

If a baby is born with the umbilical cord wrapped around their wrist or in their hand, the baby is given either the name Àìná or Òjọ́, depending on whether the child is an obìnrin or ọkùnrin, respectively. These children are believed to have a deep connection to their ancestors, since the umbilical cord represents the connection between the physical world and the ancestral plane.

Among Yoruba, Igbo, and Annang communities, women were expected to abstain from sex for one to three years. It was believed that engaging in sexual intercourse too soon after birth could endanger the child.[17] The practice of postpartum abstinence helped with birth spacing, ensuring that children received adequate attention from their mothers.

CREATING BLACK FAMILIES

In precolonial Yoruba society, the agbo ilé (family compound) was structured for the purpose of childrearing. Since children were considered blessings, producing and raising children was viewed with utmost importance and respect. Since children were seen as symbols of wealth and prosperity, mothers were seen as the harbingers of good fortune for a community. The sacredness of motherhood is represented through the many orisas that are mothers. Lineage was traditionally tracked matrilineally, and parental rights were automatically given to the birthing obìnrin. Since motherhood was held in such high regard, if a partnership didn't lead to children, an aya had the freedom to move on and seek other partnerships. For ọkùnrin to secure paternity rights, marriage to an obìnrin was required. Fatherhood did not depend on biological paternity. If an ọkọ and aya had trouble conceiving, an aya could produce a child with another member of the agbo ilé or an outsider. The ọkọ would still be considered the father under these circumstances. As long as an ọkọ was married to an aya he could secure paternity rights.[18] This is evident in the oríkì, sacred poetry, which often prescribes spiritual remedies for "wifelessness." Since ọkùnrin depended on marriage to secure paternity rights, ọkùnrin paid idaana (bride wealth) to the family of the iyawo (bride). The idaana symbolized the lifelong goods and services the groom was expected to provide to the iyawo's family. Divorce was a common practice in Yoruba society, with little stigma attached to it, another reason for the oríkì to frequently mention wifelessness.[19]

Although monogamous marriages were the norm, polygamy, the practice of one man having multiple wives, was common throughout precolonial Yoruba society. Interest in polygamy was directly connected to the importance the Yoruba community placed on childbearing.[20] Polygamous arrangements and the central living structure of agbo ilé encouraged community child-rearing practices. Division of labor among different members of the family fostered a collaborative environment. Responsibilities related to cooking and child care were distributed among the ọkọ and aya of the agbo ilé on a seniority basis. Children and newer aya cooked and were responsible for many of the child-rearing responsibilities, while more senior aya and ọkọ, regardless of gender, worked on the family trade, worked in the market, or farmed. Though Oyèrónkẹ́ argues that polygamy had benefits for both the ọkọ and aya, polygamy remains a highly controversial practice.

BLACK FAMILY "DYSFUNCTION" AND THE ROLE OF MOTHERHOOD

Motherhood is a controversial and contentious topic within the political context of the United States. Women's autonomy when it comes to family planning continues to be under attack in the West in the form of anti-abortion laws and abstinence-only sex education. Multiple factors both push and discourage women and birthing people to have children, creating a cycle fueled by lack of social support and resources. For Black women in particular, motherhood has been a fraught topic.

In *Killing the Black Body*, Dorothy E. Roberts explores the history of Black women's fight for reproductive justice. Stereotypes about Black women inform the way society views Black motherhood and frames the conversation about what reproductive justice means for Black women. The "Jezebel" stereotype, which paints Black women as promiscuous seductresses, follows Black women into motherhood, painting them as irresponsible and indiscriminate mothers. While the Jezebel stereotype paints Black women as hypersexual, the "Mammy" stereotype imagines them as asexual, submissive caretakers. The image of the Mammy is based on her role as a servant to white families, providing all types of domestic labor, including cooking, cleaning, and child care. The Mammy represented the ideal Black woman; she was devoted to her white employers and praised for her selfless and caring nature. As Roberts explains, "the ideology of the Mammy placed no value on Black women as the mothers of their own children."[21] Her time spent caring for the children of white families meant that she was unable to provide that care to her own children.

Throughout history, Black women's right to motherhood and the right to reproductive autonomy have been challenged. As a result of chattel slavery, Black mothers had no legal claim to their children. Enslaved women were extremely valuable to their masters for both their labor and their ability to bear children. The law made it such that enslaved women's children were the property of her master. Enslavers could increase their wealth by controlling the reproductive capacity of enslaved women.[22] When the transport of slaves was outlawed in 1808 in the United States, reproduction was the main way to increase the population of enslaved people. To take control over their reproduction, enslaved women induced abortions through a variety of techniques. Though herbally induced abortions were the most common, enslaved women also used "violent exercise" and "external and internal manipulation." At times, midwives conspired with pregnant enslaved women to help induce and cover up abortions.

Sociologists of the late nineteenth and twentieth centuries published report after report about the supposed dysfunction of Black family life. Linking the matriarchal structure of many Black families to the residual effects of enslavement was a central theme of many of these reports. In *Wayward Lives, Beautiful Experiments,* Saidiya Hartman analyzes the reports written by W. E. B. Du Bois and his intellectual counterparts at the turn of the twentieth century. In his reports, Du Bois blamed the dysfunction of the Black family on "lax morals, promiscuity, children born out of wedlock, and the disregard for marriage."[23] He believed that holdovers from enslavement and city life conspired to lead to the social crisis plaguing the Black family. To Du Bois, "cohabitation was a direct offshoot of plantation life."[24] Du Bois and his contemporaries viewed the high number of unmarried women in cities as part of the problem. According to them, unmarried women meant lowered standards of living and "fostered casual relations, cohabitation, [and] the taking up and casting off of lovers at will."[25]

Du Bois's concerns about the state of the Black family were far from unique. While he acknowledged the brilliance and ingenuity of Black people alongside his harsh critiques, white sociologists tended to paint Black Americans as a monolith plagued by poverty and loose morals. Sociologists both before and after Du Bois have claimed that the Black family's dysfunction is an ingrained part of Black identity. Some sociologists point to the aftermath of slavery while others claimed it was biological or cultural conditions that predisposed Black people to familial dysfunction. In "Mama's Baby, Papa's Maybe: An American Grammar Book," Hortense Spillers discusses the infamous Moynihan Report written by former US Senator Daniel Patrick Moynihan. Titled *The Negro Family: The Case for National Action,* Moynihan argues that the structure of the Black family lies at the center of the widening inequality gap between Black and white Americans.

Moynihan states that "the Negro family in the urban ghettos is crumbling" and that it poses a threat to the nation as a whole. He argues that "a national effort is required" and that the federal government should focus its efforts toward "the establishment of a stable Negro family structure." Moynihan claims that the matriarchal structures found within Black families "seriously retards the progress of the group as a whole, and imposes a crushing burden on the Negro male and, in consequence, on a great many Negro women as well."[26] While Moynihan admits that there is no reason why a male-headed household is inherently better, he argues that it's detrimental for Black families to practice a family structure different from dominant white society. Moynihan and other sociologists place the blame of the Black family's dysfunction on Black women. The "dominance" and "strength" of Black women becomes a "pathology" that emasculates Black men and undermines Black femininity in the eyes of the West.[27]

All of these sociologists failed to adequately contextualize the impact of over 250 years of destabilization, generational trauma, displacement, and violence that marked the transatlantic slave trade. Their hypotheses about the Black family and Black motherhood rarely began with "the arrival of twenty-odd Africans in Jamestown, Virginia."[28] As both Spillers and Hartman point out, the historical archive lacks information about the treatment of captive African women during the Middle Passage. Spillers argues that the Middle Passage served as the point of sociopolitical transformation that led to "ungendering" of African women. The early cargo records often lacked clear gender identifiers, referring to captive Africans as quantities. This ungendering gave way to deprivation of maternal rights from Black and African women. The violence of enslavement deprived Black women of motherhood, creating a system that controlled Black women's bodies and their children, stripping them of their autonomy. Enslaved women's reproduction was governed by crop cycles. Children were typically born in late summer and early fall. This implies that conception occurred sometime during November, December, or January, when labor requirements were lower due to the harsh winter conditions.[29] The seasonality of conception led to increased infant mortality rates. Late summer and early fall birth coincided with the harvest season, the most labor-intensive time of the year.

Enslaved women were deprived of the opportunity to nurture their own children. Mothers were forced to leave their nursing and other young children at home for hours while they worked in the fields. Enslaved people that were too weak, too old, or too young often watched young children while their mothers worked. When possible, enslaved women developed ingenious ways to care for their children while working in the fields. They sometimes tied their children to their backs or dug shallow holes to lay them in.[30]

With legal claim to their children, enslavers had full control of the familial structure of Black families. Families were torn apart at slave auctions. Relatives were sold to different plantations, never to be seen again. Children were sold or apprenticed out, sometimes for as long as ten years.[31] Enslavers also weaponized children against their mothers. To prevent enslaved women from running away, enslavers used children as hostages to lure escaped women back to the plantation. Unwilling to leave their children, women often hid in nearby swamps and marshes for stretches of time before returning to the plantation. The bond between mother and child resulted in more men fleeing slavery than women. The average runaway was a lone man between the ages of sixteen and thirty-five who was forced to leave his family behind.[32]

The arguments surrounding the supposed dysfunction of Black families is rooted in a belief of a universal nuclear family, based on white, upwardly-mobile families and rooted in gender norms, patriarchy, and capitalism. Prior to the industrial revolution, most white people lived in large extended family networks, typically centered around farming. It was common for a house to include grandparents, cousins, uncles, and aunts as well as the extended workforce of servants and enslaved people.[33] After the Industrial Revolution, more people began moving to cities in search of new opportunities, shifting the family structure in the process. For Black Southerners, the search for opportunity up North while fleeing racist violence was termed the Great Migration. Some families doubled down, holding tight to their extended family networks in an era marked by shifting attitudes. Other families began to become more and more fragmented as young people fled rural areas for bustling urban cities. This coincided with the influx of immigrants from Eastern Europe who began moving to the United States in the late 1800s, fleeing harsh economic conditions.

As more people moved to cities, the average age of marriage began to drop for urban men and women. The families these young couples started were nuclear families, made up of a male breadwinner, a wife who sometimes held gendered jobs outside the home but whose typical sphere was the household, and a few kids.[34] The nuclear family entered its renaissance between 1950 and 1965, when wages increased, union membership was high, and home convenience inventions took off. In his 1964 report Moynihan states, "The white family has achieved a high degree of stability and is maintaining that stability."[35] The short-lived success of the nuclear family imprinted an almost unshakeable image into the American psyche of what a successful family looked like in the modern era. In the years that followed, the nuclear family began to break apart as capitalism continued to push people toward individualism and isolation.

The nuclear family's pervasiveness in Western culture can be felt in the structure of homes and apartments that are designed for a privatized existence.[36] As wages began to decrease and union membership dropped, families under economic pressure started falling apart. The nuclear family model works extremely well for wealthy families who are able to outsource child care and housework while reaping the economic benefits of caring for a limited number of people. For everyone else, nuclear families intensify the already complex interpersonal relationships that make up families. In *Abolish the Family*, Sophie Lewis argues that the crushing unaffordability of raising children in the West combined with the gendered and racialized division of labor within the household creates an environment ripe for conflict and abuse. The nuclear family has failed to provide many people with the care and support they need. Lewis argues that the nuclear family structure functions as a replacement for community care and a tool for capitalist production. Confining people to one set definition of family limits our imagination and prevents people from fostering supportive relationships outside the traditional nuclear structure. It's not surprising that many people find themselves having complicated and fraught relationships with their families.[37]

I spent most of 2020 working as a confidential youth advocate for housing and food-insecure youth at a domestic violence shelter in Portland, Oregon. My job was to help youth navigate difficult situations without all the requirements of being a mandatory reporter. Oftentimes, youth experience violence from parents or relatives that is only exacerbated if law enforcement or child protective services are involved without regard to the complexities of the youth's family structure. Though my job was incredibly stressful, it felt rewarding to advocate for youth autonomy. Many of the youth I worked with had family members who perpetuated harm against them, making it difficult for them to seek access to care. In these instances, mandatory reporting often exacerbated problems at home, with children receiving retaliatory backlash from parents who have received child abuse or neglect inquiries. Just as Lewis argues, the nuclear family failed to provide the care my youth clients deserved. It left them isolated with few options for alternative care that wasn't youth shelters or foster care. My youth advocacy work opened my eyes to the important fight for children's rights and autonomy. Until children's rights are firmly secured, the familial structure has to be reimagined to ensure that children receive adequate love and care.

Family is the first environment children enter. As the basic social organizing unit, family acts as a microcosm of society at large. So many people are raised in families with tense dynamics that lead to generational trauma. The transatlantic slave trade, chattel slavery, white supremacy, displacement, and racism left such strong lasting impacts on our ancestors that the evidence is embedded in our DNA. The trauma of enslavement spills over into our familial relationships, leading some of us to replicate oppressive systems within our homes. In the first chapter of *All About Love*, bell hooks explains that love and abuse are two forces that cannot coexist. Love, as bell hooks defines it, is an action composed of care, affection, responsibility, respect, commitment, and trust.[38] hooks recounts her own experience of corporal punishment at the hands of her parents. Spanking or whipping were common practices in many Black families. My grandmother told stories about her mother's punishments, which often involved spankings with a switch, a small tree branch. As a child, I was spanked by parents but never by any of my other relatives. Though I wasn't spanked often, I have vivid memories of spankings involving rulers and belts. Scholars argue that the trauma of enslavement and the European notion that children are born sinful influence Black parenting practices.[39] hooks argues that if we would not tolerate corporal punishment between adults, we should not tolerate it when it comes to children. She argues that it's crucial that we develop ways to offer loving discipline to children who are denied full rights in our society.[40] A younger generation of Black parents are turning to gentle parenting approaches to raise children. Gentle parenting is an approach to child-rearing that focuses on affirming children's feelings and emotions. Gentle parenting is not without discipline; it just looks different than corporal punishment. Discipline is framed as teaching moments, requiring parents to be patient and learn skills for regulating their emotions. Gentle parenting requires both parents and children to learn skills that build emotional intelligence.

As Lewis argues, a revolutionary approach to familial structures requires an openness to challenges and critiques from all members of the family, including children. Children have their own unique ways of relating that give way to perspectives on relationships that challenge hierarchical and patriarchal familial structures. Revolutionary ideals that challenge the existing notions of the family require input from people who traditionally hold marginalized positions within the heteronormative patriarchal family.

ALTERNATIVE FAMILY STRUCTURES

Despite the trauma of slavery, Black people fought to keep their families together. Free Black people often bought their relatives' freedom when possible. Enslaved people managed to create intimate family structures dependent on communal care and kinship. Since couples were often separated, households made up of women and children were more common among enslaved people than their white counterparts. Since the family unit could be torn apart at any moment, enslaved communities "created networks of mutual obligation that reached beyond the nuclear family."[41] It was common practice for children to address all Black adults as "Uncle" or "Aunt" as both a sign of respect and a symbol of familial relationship among non–blood relatives. The strength of the families and communities that enslaved Africans created is in their adaptability, acceptance, and communal systems of care.

In Haiti, communities known as *lakou* formed as anti-plantation living compounds. Centered around the concept of autonomy, the lakou prioritizes self-reliance through an agricultural model.[42] The structure of the lakou was a cluster of houses encircling a large plot of land. The lakou functioned as a safeguard against the return of the plantation, functioning as an egalitarian system outside the state. A lakou is created when a founding ancestor settles on a plot of land and raises a family. The land is then passed down to the children, with sons and daughters inheriting the land equally. Children were raised communally by all members of the lakou. Each child had a personal stake in the communal land. At birth, children's umbilical cords were buried on the land. A fruit tree would be planted at the umbilical cord's burial site. The fruit tree acts as a "trust fund" for the child, providing sustenance in the form of fruit that could be eaten or sold. Within the lakou, a decentralized ownership model is practiced to ensure that the land is not consolidated under a single owner.

The emphasis on self-reliance made wage labor undesirable for members of the lakou. Wage labor requires workers to work for the benefit of their employers, not themselves. Rural Haitians gave up or forwent salaried labor, viewed as the enemy of autonomy, in favor of communal agricultural work.

In Vodou, the lakou plays a central role. The compound provides practitioners with a direct connection to the land of their ancestors. Communal cemeteries are established within the lakou, serving as a constant reminder of the community's connection to the ancestors.

Historically, Black families faced significant economic disadvantages compared to their white counterparts. At the turn of the century, about a third of Black urban residents were domestic laborers. Nine out of ten women were domestic laborers, working as cooks, housekeepers, laundresses, and nannies.[43] Forced into meager housing while doing degrading jobs that raised the question of whether or not slavery had actually ended, Black people protested against oppression wherever they could. They reimagined family and relations by forming relationships and families that broke the standard mold: households run by mothers, aunts, and grandmother, fleeting and casual romantic relationships, and interracial relationships with the Jewish residents of their community. The communities and ways of living that Black Americans created were both a survival strategy and a rebellion. Saidiya Hartman argues that the so-called dysfunction of the Black family that sociologists railed against is simply a strategy for survival rooted in "flexible and elastic kinship" and "the generosity and mutuality of the poor." Through what she describes as "an attempt to elude capture by never settling" by using "the ex-slave's fugitive gestures," Black Americans imagine a way to move through city life that afforded them as much freedom as possible.[44]

In *Joyful Militancy,* carla bergman and Nick Montgomery argue that "freedom and friendship used to mean the same thing: intimate, interdependent relationships and the commitment to face the world together."[45] They argue that it is the interconnected relationships we form with each other and the world around us that make us feel free, not the isolationism pushed onto us by capitalism. Individualism breeds fear through social isolation and mistrust. Nina Simone's assertion that freedom is that absence of fear serves as a reminder to seek systems that reduce anxiety and bring us closer to a sense of inner peace. The communal living of Black people across the diaspora creates neighborhoods, families, and communities founded in a sense of mutual care. The mutual care of interconnected communities reduces fear as people build trust with their neighbors.

Black families have had to find ways to care for each other in spite of the oppressive forces that wish to separate us. The mass incarceration of Black people has torn families apart, forcing Black people to create adaptive structures to maintain family relationships. According to the Federal Bureau of Prisons, Black people are disproportionately represented in the prison population, accounting for 38 percent of inmates.[46] In *Somebody's Daughter,* Ashley C. Ford recounts the ways her father's incarceration impacted her relationship with him as well as her mother and grandmother when she was growing up.[47] The absence of Ford's father required that her family adapt, creating a multigenerational structure led by her mother and grandmother.

In his 1992 book *Climbing Jacob's Ladder: The Enduring Legacy of African-American Families,* Andrew Billingsley discusses the ways Black families have adapted to economic, social, and spiritual demands by creating a variety of family structures to survive. He discusses the high rate of informal adoption among Black families by extended family members like grandparents and aunts. Both of my paternal grandparents were adopted, my grandfather Lawrence by his aunt and uncle after his parents passed away, and my grandmother Sandra by her biological mother's close friend. Grandparents are the main caretakers of adopted children, forming multigenerational family units. The 1989 US Census reported that 1.2 million Black children lived with their grandparents.[48] A 2022 Pew Research study found that 26 percent of Black Americans lived in multigenerational households compared to 13 percent of white Americans.[49] For most of my childhood, my grandmother Louise split her time between living with my family in Orange County and her Los Angeles home. Since both my parents worked, she co-raised my brother and me alongside my parents. My mother was a schoolteacher in a different school district than the one my brother and I attended, so our school breaks didn't always line up. When she wasn't available to watch my brother and me, we spent our evenings and summer breaks at my aunt's house. We were raised through the care of my parents, grandmother, and aunt, rarely spending time in afterschool care or day care.

Black families are also built on extended kin networks, made of non–blood relatives. Affectionately referred to as "play cousins," many Black children have close familial relationships with each other as a result of their parents' friendships. "Play mothers," "play aunts," and "play uncles" refer to the family-like dynamics formed between the non–blood relative adults. As a young child, I grew up with the children of my parents' close family friends. Many of my earliest childhood memories were of playing with the daughters of my parents' friends. Their parents feel like distant aunts and uncles to me because of their consistent presence during the formative years of my life. Though we're all grown up now, our parents remain close, sending holiday cards back and forth and attending birthday parties.

Billingsley describes three main types of Black families: the nuclear family, the extended family, and the augmented family, which he defines as families made up of blood relatives and non–blood relatives living within the same household. He also explores the diversity of Black family structures, which include couples living together without children and blended families made up of stepparents and stepchildren. Through blood relatives and kinship networks, Black people have found ways to create loving support systems. The diversity of Black family structures is a testament to the adaptability and resilience of Black people.

CONCLUSION

Reimagining family life outside the constraints of capitalism, heteronormativity, and the nuclear family requires a radical imagination and the bravery to chart your own path. Looking to our ancestors for guidance, we remind ourselves that other ways for building families and raising children are possible.

Children are mirrors that reflect the past, present, and future back to us. They bring blessings and lessons from their ancestors with them when they are born into this world. They serve as guidance and reminders to center play and joy in our lives. Through our children, we learn how to build loving relationships and how to exercise patience. The lessons we teach them within the families we create shape the collective future of the world.

Building a supportive environment begins with building a world where Black women and mothers are respected and honored. Undoing generations of medical racism and eugenics requires us to center Black women's lived experiences in the medical field and beyond. We are experts of our own bodies.

We deserve safe and loving communities to raise our children and form families. Time and time again history has shown us that the key to a thriving community is mutual aid and community care. Challenging the nuclear family is not about rejecting any family systems that resemble it. It is about creating alternatives to "the spatial division of people through suburbanization, incarceration, schooling, dispossession, and displacement."[50]

Experimentation is the key to creating something new. When the forces of capitalism, white supremacy, and patriarchy push us to our limits, there is no other option besides rebellion. Rebellion and protest come in many forms—sometimes the most powerful are in the small everyday acts where we decide to take a different path. We can divest from the systems and structures that harm us by building new ones within our families. We can plant the seeds of social change by creating the world we wish to live in through our relationships with our loved ones and our community.

5

THE BLESSING OF ÌṢẸ́GUN

Those who want to kill me will be destroyed; they will go down to the depths of the earth. They will be given over to the sword and become food for jackals.
—PSALM 63:9–10

The cruelties of property and privilege are always more ferocious than the revenges of poverty and oppression.
—C. L. R. JAMES, *THE BLACK JACOBINS*

It wasn't unusual to go through extended periods of time where I felt generally depressed and disinterested in things that normally brought me joy. These episodes would creep up slowly, and then gradually the bad day turned into a bad week, and before I knew it a bad two or three months. I would feel tired, irritable, aimless, and always dissatisfied.

But when I began to feel similar shifts in my mood in late 2021, something about it felt different. Throughout all the other waves of depression I managed to maintain a small but enduring amount of motivation. I used my personal goals as the guiding force, and I hoped that by accomplishing my goals the cloud of melancholy would lift. This time, I no longer felt I had any tangible goals left to accomplish. I had finished grad school and was working at a nonprofit as a DEI educator. I had once imagined that teaching people about race, class, and world history would be a dream job. Now that seemed silly, and I felt drained and aimless.

I didn't realize at the time that this was brought on by overwhelming burnout. I'd struggled through the onset of the pandemic and the Trumpian political atmosphere, leading workshops and trainings about implicit bias and white privilege. Each session I led made me feel more and more discouraged. I spent hours shifting through depressing information about anti-Blackness, homophobia, anti-Indigeneity, and ableism, searching for examples I could use in my slide decks. I received very little training or support from my organization on how to approach sensitive topics and work with diverse clients, who left workshops either very appreciative or very upset. Most of my workshops were held virtually, and at the end of every session I walked away from the computer covered in sweat from head to toe. Everything I did felt futile and pointless.

I walked away from that period of my life with a lot of cynicism around DEI workshops. Working within a capitalistic system was never going to create the path toward collective liberation I was so adamantly fighting for. Clients hired my organization because it was "politically trendy" (or good for business) to engage with organizations that led inclusivity workshops and trainings. The burnout I felt came from a very real understanding that the fight for liberation wasn't futile but the tactic I was using was. It was made worse by the fact that my livelihood depended on me getting up and leading these workshops no matter how badly I wanted to do anything other than work.

Over time I've come to understand that I went through an experience similar to what a lot of people new to activism go through. There's initially so much joy and excitement and ego attached to the ways many people approach activism or community work fueled by a deep desire to "change the world." It's easy to read a few books, attend a few protests or community-centered events, and feel energized. It's only once the work has begun that you start to realize how insurmountable the forces of white supremacy, capitalism, and patriarchy begin to feel.

So many brilliant theorists and organizers emphasize the importance of joy and resilience because they know how disheartening and all-consuming this work can be. Oftentimes, the approaches that many young organizers and activists adopt aren't effective or are rendered ineffective by the larger systems they're operating under. Universities and nonprofits are often the first institutions young activists find themselves in. While both places can be a source for learning and community building, it quickly becomes apparent that the forces of bureaucracy and capitalism quell honest attempts at radical change. When your livelihood and education are tied to these institutions, it makes it harder to push against those forces and even harder to leave.

I don't claim to have answers about the best ways to organize or how to build community. I don't identify as an activist or an organizer. I've learned over the years to lean into my strengths while supporting and uplifting people who are stronger in areas I am not. I'm a learner, and my area of expertise lies in my passion for reading and intense curiosity. Later in 2021, I refocused my energy, and instead of trying to dream up ways to dismantle global systems of oppression, I focused my attention on my community. It sounds cliché, but I began with simply making friends and building stronger connections with people locally who were dedicated and passionate about the same sociopolitical issues I'm passionate about. I also began studying history differently. I stopped inundating myself with information about events highlighting the atrocities committed in the name of "god, glory, and gold" that left me feeling angry and overwhelmed.

I began trying to balance the painful and tragic histories and present atrocities with stories of small victories that serve as both a beacon of hope and tools for imagining different futures. Which brings us to this chapter: the last of the five core blessings in Ifá is Ire Ìṣẹ́gun, the blessing of victory.

The path toward liberation is not linear. Victory does not mean the entire battle is won. Victories typically look like the gradual shift in attitudes or moments that pave the way for larger movements to take hold.

OVERCOMING NEGATIVE FORCES

Though it comes last, victory is one of the most vital concepts in the tradition. All of the other blessings build off each other, each one laying the foundation for the next. Victory functions a bit differently. While the blessings of àìkú, àjé, ọkọ/aya, and ọmọ all lay the foundation for one to be victorious, victory is also a necessary component for achieving all the blessings that proceed it.

Ire Ìṣẹ́gun is described as the blessing of being victorious over negative forces. Just as there are core blessings, there are core negative forces as well. Known as *osogbo, ibi,* or *ajogun,* these forces are a daily part of everyday life. Based on the teachings from my ilé, there are five main negative forces: *iku* (death), *aro* (sickness), *ofo* (loss), *ija* (fight or contention), and *oran* (unforeseen negative forces). Some ilés focus on the first four, leaving off oran. Through divination, *ebo* (sacrifice), herbalism, and maintaining *iwa pele* (good character or having a cool head), practitioners aim to avert negative forces.

Victory is only achieved by warding off each of the negative forces. To achieve Ire Àìkú, the blessing of longevity, you have to be victorious over the negative forces of iku and aro. Maintaining wealth requires continuous victory over the negative force of ofo. Lasting partnership requires victory over the negative force of ija. Without victory at every stage, none of the previous blessings would be possible. Negative spiritual forces can attach themselves to an individual or to a family, creating "generational curses" that continue to plague families for generations unless broken. If a family continuously fights across generations or has trouble maintaining wealth across generations, that family may be plagued by the spirit of ija or ofo.

In Ifá cosmology, everything has a spiritual root or an underlying spiritual explanation. The ajogun represent the underlying spiritual forces behind death, illness, loss, and conflict. To adequately address any negativity a devotee may be experiencing, the spiritual components must be addressed first. During divination, the ire and osogbo (ajogun) of the devotee is determined. Typically, cowrie shells represent ire and bones represent osogbo. During divination, the babalawo or iyanifa will periodically clear the markings off the board with either cowrie shells or bone, depending on the ire or osogbo determined during the divination process. African American spiritual traditions also believe that illness, death, and misfortune often have spiritual roots. Sudden ailments, misfortune, or radical shifts in behavior were believed to be caused by conjure harming, the use of spiritual power, and herbal knowledge to cause harm.[1] In Ifá and other ATRs and ADRs, calling upon spiritual forces for protection is a central part of self-defense against spiritual and physical enemies. Esu, Ṣàngó, and Egun are three forces that are essential to the concept of victory. They represent communication, battle, and tradition, respectively. The most successful victories in Black diasporic history expertly combine all three concepts to strategically organize mass uprising, protests, and slave revolts.

VICTORIES AGAINST CAPITALISM

Ṣàngó is the orisa of fire, thunder, lightning, and battle. Like many other orisas, Ṣàngó's attributes are connected to both spiritual concepts and the life of a deified ruler of Oyo, Nigeria. As the ruler of Oyo, Ṣàngó was known as a fierce warrior and leader, feared for his prowess in battle and his temper; myths spoke of his spiritual and militaristic power. Ṣàngó is also referred to as Jakuta, which translates to "the one who fights with stones." Many scholars believe Jakuta was the original name of the orisa of thunder and lightning but was absorbed as a second name for Ṣàngó when Ṣàngó the ruler was deified.[2]

Ṣàngó/Jakuta represents the rage of Olódùmarè and is often associated with hot-tempered men throughout the diaspora. Although Ṣàngó embodies a strong masculine force, like many orisa, aspects of his personality are associated with gender play. In one myth, Ọya, Ṣàngó's wife, cuts off her braids and gives them to Ṣàngó along with her clothes to allow him to escape the enemy. Devotees who have been "mounted" by Ṣàngó dance in ways that emphasize Ṣàngó's masculine and feminine qualities. It's also common for devotees of Ṣàngó to braid their hair in more traditionally feminine styles as a nod to the Ọya hair myth.

Due to his reputation as a warrior, Ṣàngó is the orisa that assists practitioners in being victorious over negative forces, leading to his widespread popularity across the diaspora. Ṣàngó's connection to fire represents his creative, destructive, and purifying nature. Victory requires both creativity and destruction. Creativity is required to imagine new futures, organize groups of people for mass protests, and strategize militaristically. Destruction is a necessary and unavoidable part of decolonization. For new systems to be built, the old ones have to be destroyed. Ṣàngó encourages us to connect to the energy of fire as we prepare for battle.

Self-defense is a central component of ATRs and ADRs, both spiritually and physically. Spiritual defenses range from protecting your energy after initiation ceremonies or other spiritually significant periods to using spiritual tools to defend against outside forces. White supremacy wages economic, mental, physical, and spiritual war against indigenous peoples globally. The loss of African and Indigenous spiritual knowledge is a core tactic used by white supremacy to keep people disconnected from their traditional ways of healing, connection, and protection. As I mentioned in chapter 1, Ifá and other indigenous traditions are nature-based practices that incorporate the use of plants and medicinal herbs for both spiritual and physical well-being. When we are disconnected from ancestral knowledge, we're forced to out-source our physical, mental, and spiritual health by seeking knowledge outside our communities. Not only does this result in us using systems that are not culturally relevant, it reinforces internalized concepts of inferiority by reinforcing narratives that center Western systems of knowing.

Afro-Indigenous spiritual self-defense consists of protection, healing or cleansing, and defense. Protection rituals and charms work either physically, spiritually, or psychically. For example, after taking spiritual baths, following an orí appeasement, or during stressful situations, it's a common practice to cover your head with a scarf or head wrap. Keeping the head covered is a way to protect yourself during a vulnerable psychic state when you may be more sensitive to outside influence. In the US South, among rootworkers and conjurers, sacred African chants for protection were replaced by Bible verses. The book of Psalms is widely used by rootworkers for incantations used to ward off evil, attract love, and usher in wealth and prosperity. Psalms and other sections of the Bible were commonly used in hoodoo practices because of a belief in the spiritual power of most sacred texts. Enslaved Africans believed in the power of the Bible and incorporated it into traditional practices to imbue them with added potency or to replace indigenous prayers or oríkì that were lost with time.

Other methods for spiritual protection involve herbs and talismans. High John the Conqueror root (*Ipomoea purga*) is famously used among hoodoo rootworkers and incorporated into mojo bags, sewn into clothes, or carried in pockets for protection. Devil's shoestring (*Tephrosia virginiana*) and asafetida (dried latex from *Ferula* roots) are common herbs used in protection rituals and charms to ward off evil. Spiritual herbs are incorporated into spiritual baths, soaps, and floor washes to cleanse, protect, ward off evil, or usher in good luck. They're also incorporated into talismans and charms that the user carries on them or places in specified locations. Originating from Kongo, *nkisi* (plural *minkisi*) are ritual objects imbued with otherworldly power. Feathers, bones, herbs and other materials are incorporated into the construction of an nkisi, typically prepared by skilled *nganga*, Kikongo priests, and sacred healers. Some minkisi were used for healing, while others caused illness or aided in determining the innocence or guilt of accused criminals.[3] Raffia bags or wooden sculptures were used to house the spirit of the nkisi. Kongolese cosmology also regarded illnesses and misfortunes as having roots in the spiritual realm. Minkisi were used to intervene in these spiritual matters.

In Kikongo spirituality, the *kindoki,* or spiritual force required to exercise ritual powers, is similar to the concept of asé in Yoruba spirituality. Kindoki is the necessary force and violence required to alter the physical and metaphysical realms. Through the use of kindoki, trained nganga harness the spiritual power that resides with minkisi during rituals. Minkisi made of animal skins or raffia bags were filled with medicinal objects, selected for their metaphysical properties rather than pharmacological ones, and tied with string or cord to symbolize the control and submission of the inhabiting spirit.[4] This class of minkisi were the precursors to Haitian *pakèt kongo* and hoodoo mojo bags.

Both Haitian pakèt kongo and hoodoo mojo bags are used for protection and healing. Pakèt kongo are used to activate the lwa and serve as a physical contact point where the power of a particular lwa can be accessed. Mojo bags, also called *gris-gris* bags, mojo hands, or conjure bags, are amulets made of clothes filled with herbs, crystals, or other spiritual objects for protection, luck, and healing. A common use of mojo bags was for luck by frequent gamblers, sometimes referred to as their lucky hand. Wooden minkisi were carved in the shape of humans or animals with a small opening carved into the stomach where medicinal objects were placed. Red- and white-colored objects and pigments were commonly used in the construction of minkisi. In Kongo cosmology, white represents the land of the dead while red represents the liminal space between the physical and spiritual realm.

The objects placed inside minkisi had metonymic and metaphorical importance. For example, stones may be included in an nkisi intended to remove a tumor, while feathers may be included in an nkisi used to seek out information or seek out a wrongdoer. The items placed within minkisi served a variety of purposes, including healing, harming, or evoking desire. Including a *tonda* (mushroom) in a nkisi intended to invoke desire was used as a Kikongo pun on the term *tondwa*, which means "to desire."[5] Personal effects such as hair or fingernails were included in minkisi to identify the intended victim. A common hoodoo and African American practice is burning hair after receiving a haircut to ensure that no one with ill intent is able to get hold of your personal effects. To arouse the spirit within the nkisi, the nganga would traditionally bang, shake, or strike the nkisi. After the colonization of Kongo by Portuguese slave traders, methods for invoking the spirit within the nkisi shifted from banging in favor of driving nails into the body of wooden nkisi. Around the eighteenth century, driving nails into minkisi became the primary method for invoking the spirit due to the association between nails and the Christian crucifix.[6] The symbol of Christ nailed to the cross resonated with Kikongo notions of awakening spiritual power. The minkisi produced during this period were visually stunning. The nailed minkisi were the precursors to voodoo dolls used primarily to curse or harm the intended victim.

VICTORIES AGAINST CAPTIVITY

Slave revolts always invoke images of violent uprisings against colonialism, capitalism, and white supremacy. At their core, slave revolts are an attempt at regaining autonomy through decolonization. When studying the history of famous uprisings led by enslaved Africans in the United States and the Caribbean, I found that African spirituality played a crucial role in many of them. Oaths were a crucial element of building solidarity and ensuring trust among revolting enslaved Africans. Oath rituals were performed as a prelude to rebellion and often incorporated elements of obeah, a broad term describing African diasporic Caribbean traditions. Prior to a 1736 rebellion in Antigua and a 1760 rebellion in Jamaica, elaborate oath rituals were performed, including elements of animal sacrifice and blood oaths.[7]

In *Mules and Men*, Zora Neale Hurston describes her hoodoo initiation led by Luke Turner, the alleged nephew of famous voodoo priestess Marie Leveau. Marie Leveau (whose last name has several alternate spellings) was known as a powerful voodoo practitioner in 1800s Louisiana. Myths about her apparent power and skill vary widely, but many claim that she had the power to both cure and curse. Turner's alleged association with Marie Leveau amplified his reputation as a hoodoo-voodoo practitioner.[8] In preparation for the initiation ceremony, Luke instructed Zora to fast for several days. The initiation involved a naming ceremony where Zora received the name Rain-Bringer, given to Luke in a message from spirit.

The ceremony culminated in a blood oath. Luke cut Zora's pinky finger and caught the gushing blood in a wine glass. He mixed the blood and wine together, and then Luke, along with five other spiritual leaders, cut their hands and mixed their blood and wine into a different glass. Zora drank from the glass with all the spiritual leaders' blood while Luke and the spiritual leaders drank from the glass containing Zora's blood. The initiation ceremony concluded with Luke "crowning" Zora with consecrated snakeskin, followed by a celebratory feast.[9]

The blood oaths taken prior to slave rebellions harken back to the ritual "scratching" involved in Palo Mayombe initiation ceremonies. The role of blood oaths prior to slave revolts serves a similar purpose to the blood oath in Zora's initiation. Blood is an important component in ATRs and ADRs because it represents the essential life force. Both Esu and Ṣàngó are associated with the color red, which represents blood, life, and vitality in Ifá. The blood oaths taken during initiation ceremonies and before rebellions serve as a reminder of the grave importance of the undertaking the initiate and

rebels are set to embark on. Both rootworkers and insurrectionists are working closely with the realm of death. Blood oaths not only bond the oath takers
together but remind them that the energy of death surrounds their mission.

The Haitian Revolution is the most successful slave revolt in history.
Through coordinated military strategy, communication, solidarity, and
fearlessness, the enslaved people of Haiti overthrew the French colonial
regime and established the first independent Black nation in the New
World. Bois Caïman, the Vodou ceremony that occurred on the eve of the
Haitian Revolution, is probably the most famous example of the incorporation of African spirituality in resistance movements. In *The Black Jacobins,*
C. L. R. James touches on the relationship between Vodou and revolution
in Haiti. As James explains, "Voodoo was the medium of the conspiracy."[10]

On the night of August 22, 1791, the leaders of the planned revolt met
somewhere in the Morne Rouge mountains. Accounts of the Vodou ceremony that took place vary, but a central component involves ebo, or sacrifice, of a pig, after which Boukman, the Vodou high priest, gave a speech
to inspire those gathered in the forest. He opens the speech by making a
distinction between the spiritual beliefs of the Black Haitians compared to
their white oppressors. He opens by stating that "the god who created the
sun which gives us light, who rouses the waves and rules the storm" is "good
to us and orders us to revenge our wrongs," while "the god of the white
man inspires him with crime." Boukman famously encourages the listeners to "throw away the symbol of the god of the whites who has so often
caused us to weep" in favor of listening to "the voice of liberty." Following
this speech, after months of coordination, enslaved Haitians murdered their
masters and set fire to plantations across the island. The fires raged, burning sugar cane and creating smoke so thick and black that "for nearly three
weeks, the people of Le Cap could barely distinguish day from night."[11] The
Haitian Revolution would continue for several years, concluding in 1804.
Haiti became the first independent Black nation to successfully overthrow
the colonial government.

In the Americas, Christian and African spiritual influences formed
unique traditions and beliefs among enslaved Africans. Nat Turner and the
rebellion of 1831 illustrate the ways the confluence of Christian and African

practices provided the spiritual backing for several slave revolts. Growing up, Nat Turner was known for his prophetic abilities, usually brought on by a series of visions he interpreted as messages from god. Turner's religious paternal grandmother and African-born mother influenced his understanding and interpretation of religious and spiritual phenomena. Leading up to the rebellion of 1831, Turner experienced a religious epiphany following a series of visions in 1822, 1825, and 1828. Like many other enslaved Africans, Turner's version of Christianity relied heavily on communication with the spiritual realm, which is a deeply African practice.[12]

Other famous slave revolts had more explicit connections to African spiritual traditions. Denmark Vesey was a carpenter who purchased his freedom and planned one of the largest and most extensive insurrection plots among enslaved people in the Americas. Through his membership in the African Methodist Church, Vesey and his comrades secretly planned and organized an insurrection against the white residents and enslavers in Charleston, South Carolina. Vesey used religion as a motivating force, using stories from the Old Testament to draw parallels to enslaved Africans and the Israelites of the Bible to convince his comrades of the righteousness of their cause.[13]

Vesey worked closely with a conjure man named Gullah Jack, the leader of the Gullah Society, a church-based association of Black people predominantly from the Gullah community. Ethnically, the Gullah of South Carolina and the Sea Islands maintained many of their African practices, specifically Kongolese and Akan practices, due to the remote communities that formed along the Carolina coast and among the surrounding islands. Leading up to the rebellion, Gullah Jack distributed *cullah* talismans made of crab claws for invulnerability during battle and performed a ritual that incorporated verses from Psalms and the consumption of a partially raw chicken.[14]

VICTORIES AGAINST WHITE SUPREMACY

Esu is the orisa of communication, potential, and possibility and plays a crucial role in every facet of Ifá. Esu has the ability to communicate with both the "light and dark" forces in nature. He's able to carry offerings and messages to all the irunmole and all the ajogun on the practitioner's behalf. There are many different manifestations of Esu, each one representing a different aspect of his character that speaks to his ability to transform, communicate, and catalyze life.

Esu serves as the right hand to Ọ̀rúnmìlà, the voice of Olódùmarè. Ọ̀rúnmìlà is often referred to as ẹlẹ́rìí ìpín, the witness to creation, because of his role in the Yoruba creation myth. Ọ̀rúnmìlà's prophetic ability allows him to serve as the messenger of Olódùmarè. Through divination, Ọ̀rúnmìlà deciphers the nature of the universe and, based on the information acquired, doles out instructions accordingly. Ọ̀rúnmìlà supplies the message while Esu carries the message along with the offerings to the appropriate spiritual forces. The messages from Ọ̀rúnmìlà serve as a plea to a particular spiritual force on behalf of the devotee seeking divination. The offerings serve as appeasement and payment for the spiritual work required for the devotee's blessings to manifest.

Mastering your relationship with Esu means you've developed a deeper understanding of yourself, which requires a deep connection to your orí, the spiritual and mental force that exists within all of nature. According to Ifá cosmology, everything has an orí. Your orí is your own personal divinity and should be treated as such. Honoring your orí is about developing a deeper understanding of who you are. An elder in the tradition explained to me that many people come to divination ceremonies seeking guidance or clarity when they already know the answer to their problems. As the elder explained, divination is simply a tool. It's up to the practitioner to decide whether to follow through on the recommendations from the divination ceremony or not. Divination ceremonies in Ifá are not designed for everyday advice. They're meant to decipher the nature of the energies currently surrounding your life and clear any obstacles that may prevent you from emerging victoriously. Your orí is meant to guide you through the everyday ups and downs in life. Knowing yourself and being honest about your needs and desires should provide you with the necessary information to make decisions in your life. Ifá teaches us the concept of self-assurance and encourages self-confidence through the concept of orí.

White supremacy has many manifestations and works in concert with different forces. Working alongside capitalism, white supremacy seeks to disempower Black and brown communities through mental, emotional, and physical domination. Mentally, white supremacy undermines self-confidence by instilling a sense of inferiority in oppressed peoples through a combination of tactics that seek to devalue their histories, intellect, and sense of aesthetics. In *Black Skin, White Masks*, Frantz Fanon delves into the psychological torment of white supremacy and the ways it both subtly and overtly undermines the Black psyche and instills a sense of internalized inferiority. Fanon describes the inherent desire of Black people to try to disprove myths about Black inferiority, stating that "the feeling of inferiority by Blacks is especially evident in the educated Black man who is constantly trying to overcome it."[15] He goes on to give examples of assimilation and respectability politics that include wearing European clothes, using European languages, and engaging in European forms of social interaction in an attempt to elicit a feeling of equality between Black and European people. Another example of attempts at assimilation is the desire to distance oneself from African and Indigenous peoples. Fanon mentions the ways different Black diasporic communities are offended when mistaken for various African nationalities because they view themselves as "more '*évolué*' than the African—meaning he is closer to the white man."[16]

The Black Panther Party's approach to social revolution did away with respectability politics and rooted itself firmly in the political ideologies of the Black diaspora and the Global South. Founded by Huey P. Newton and Bobby Seale, the Black Panther Party sought to dismantle white supremacy by forming a global, multicultural coalition rooted in Marxist and Pan-African ideologies. As Eldridge Cleaver, the former Minister of Information of the Black Panther Party, describes, "The ideology of the Black Panther Party is the historical experience of Black people and the wisdom gained by Black people in their four-hundred-year-long struggle against the system of racist oppression and economic exploitation . . . interpreted through the prism of the Marxist-Leninist analysis by our Minister of Defense, Huey P. Newton." Cleaver stressed the importance of creating an ideology that was by Black people for Black people. Though the Black Panthers drew from "the classical principles of scientific socialism," they reinterpreted socialist ideology into a framework uniquely their own.[17]

Foundational to the ideology of the Black Panther Party was the idea of change. Though the Panthers had a core intellectual framework that drove their work, they recognized the need to remain flexible and open to new ideas and perspectives as the world shifted around them. Cleaver describes ideology as "a comprehensive definition of a status quo that takes into account both the history and the future of that status quo and serves as the social glue that holds a people together and through which a people relate to the world and other groups of people in the world."[18] Drawing from the history of Black revolutionary movements and anti-capitalist political ideology, the Panthers created an ideology that was uniquely American. By formulating a strategy that addressed the unique racist and imperialist violence of the United States, the Panthers created a political theory and praxis that addressed issues Marx failed to understand. Cleaver and Newton understood the importance of creating an ideology that spoke directly to the material experiences of Black people in the United States and throughout the colonized world. Cleaver compared adopting Marxist ideology and any European ideology as uncomfortable, saying, "It's like praying to Jesus, a White man."[19] Fanon's work provided one of the earliest examples of developing a Marxist framework that spoke directly to Black people. Huey P. Newton and Bobby Seale adapted Fanon's theories for the Black American context, birthing the ideological framework of the Black Panther Party.

Cleaver redefined Marx's lumpenproletariat as "those who have no secure relationship or vested interest in the means of production and the institutions of capitalist society," which is made up of a class of people "who have never worked and never will; who can't find a job; who are unskilled and unfit; who have been displaced by machines, automation, and cybernation, and were never 'retained or invested with new skills'; all those on welfare or receiving state aid."[20] The Black Panther Party spoke to a group of Black people, specifically those living in urban areas, who felt that the civil rights movement's ideology had been taken to its logical conclusion. The civil rights movement had successfully played a major role in defeating legal segregation and led to the Voting Rights Act of 1965 that helped enfranchise Black communities in the South. For Black communities outside the South, the civil rights movement didn't result in significant political or economic gains, leaving them feeling frustrated and in search of new tactics to address the condition of poverty, unemployment, and violence in their communities.[21] The Black Panthers offered an alternative to the integrationist approach of the civil rights movement, centered on ideas of autonomy, international organizing, and self-defense. Both Huey and Bobby used their intellectual prowess and street smarts to help them survive during young adulthood. Their personal experiences, the intellectual Black renaissance in the Bay Area and Northern California, and the political theories of Mao, Marx, and Fanon would eventually lay the foundation for the Black Panther Party. In 1967 the Black Panther Party created their Ten Point Program, part political philosophy, part list of demands, including freedom from police brutality, clothing, education, housing, and food. "We want land, bread, housing, education, clothing, justice and peace."[22]

The Black Panthers created what Huey described as "survival programs" that addressed the gaps in community care aimed at providing a temporary solution in lieu of revolution. These programs included medical clinics, food distribution, and community education. Through their free medical clinics, many of which are still in operation today, the Panthers were one of the first organizations to bring national awareness to sickle-cell anemia, a disease that primarily impacts Black communities. Their best-known program was the Free Breakfast for Children, started in West Oakland in 1968. It spread across the country as other chapters of the Black Panther Party began their own local programs. Schools, grocery stores, and restaurants pitched in to help run the program.[23]

Breaking from the aesthetic strategy of the civil rights movement led by university students and Christian organizations set the Black Panther Party apart. The leaders of the civil rights movement of the 1950s and 1960s embraced an aesthetic culture that sought to legitimize Black Americans in the eyes of white society. Protestors were often dressed in their "Sunday's best," with straight hair and conservative clothing.[24] The uniform of the civil rights movement was intended to bolster the message that Black people deserved to be treated with respect and dignity. The Black Panther Party stood out because they took a radically different approach. The Panthers' famous uniform of a black leather jacket was inspired by old blues records. When Bobby Seale saw Huey in a black leather jacket and blue shirt, something about the outfit caught Bobby's attention. The outfit reminded Bobby of the old Louis Armstrong song "Black and Blue," specifically the lyrics "What did I do to be so black and blue?" which alluded to the singer being beaten up due to racial discrimination. They decided to make the leather jacket and blue shirt part of the original Panthers uniform. The inspiration for the black beret came weeks later after Huey and Bobby watched a documentary about the French resistance to Hitler. Together the leather jacket and black beret became a symbol of the Panthers' militancy, appealing to Black radicals and scaring the police.[25]

The Black Panthers focused on emphasizing Afrocentric beauty as a symbol of nonconformity with white standards and a rejection of respectability politics. The slogan "Black is beautiful" was widely used to describe the growing movement of pride in Black art, beauty, and culture. In Agnès Varda's 1968 documentary *Black Panthers,* a young Kathleen Cleaver describes the ideology behind the afro, stating, "All of us were born with our hair like this, and we just wear it like this because it's natural." She continues, saying that Black people everywhere are waking up to the idea that "their own natural appearance, physical appearance, is beautiful."[26] The "Black is beautiful" movement of the 1960s and 1970s focused on addressing colorism, texturism, and featurism by uplifting and embracing the diversity of beauty within the Black community. Photojournalist Kwame Brathwaite's 1962 fashion show in Harlem marked the beginning of the movement. Titled "Naturally '62," it showcased darker skin models with natural hair wearing clothing inspired by fashion in Nairobi, Lagos, and Accra.[27] Brathwaite's photos captured the changing social and cultural dynamics of the time. His images of popular artists like Bob Marley and Stevie Wonder gave context to the Black is Beautiful movement, launching it into the mainstream. As a core part of the Black Panther's aesthetic, the afro became a key symbol of Black resistance. Afros embraced natural Black hair and visually defied Eurocentric beauty standards. World-renowned artist Nina Simone, whose music became the soundtrack of the Black power movement, wore natural hair and wore clothing made of African textiles.

VICTORIES AGAINST DISCONNECTION

As I mentioned in chapter 1, ancestral veneration forms the foundational basis of ATRs and ADRs. Egun represents our genetic, cultural, and spiritual connection to the past. Ancestors are important because they hold the key to the past, which can help us better shape our futures. Ancestral veneration goes beyond simply leaving offerings for ancestors. It also involves studying the lives of our familial and collective ancestors to better understand the knowledge and wisdom they acquired during their time on earth. Ancestral veneration grounds us in our traditions and cultures, providing a tangible anchor to our past through teachings that transcend generations.

Since the transatlantic slave trade, displaced Africans have fought hard to maintain their spiritual and cultural traditions. African diasporic traditions such as Candomblé, Palo Mayombe, and hoodoo represent the ways African spiritual practices were maintained and reimagined. Centuries of stigma and persecution pushed many of these traditions underground. The stigma surrounding ATRs and ADRs is rooted in anti-Blackness. Historical narratives about African traditions associate them with "devil worship," labeling them as dark and evil, misrepresenting the tools and rituals involved in African spiritual practices. Sometimes referred to as "fetish," deriving from the Portuguese word *feitiço,* which refers to sorcery and magical arts, these spiritual items link directly back to West and West-Central African protection rituals. *Fetish* has always been used as a derogatory term to describe pagan and indigenous practices that fell outside the Catholic Church. The earliest use of the term *fetish* was to denounce the ritualistic folk practices and traditions of Europeans. Beginning in the fifteenth and sixteenth centuries, the Portuguese began referring to West African ritual objects as "feitiço." For the West, *fetish* was used as proof of European intellectual and spiritual superiority. African and Indigenous spiritual and cultural traditions have historically been viewed as appendages of the past by the West. Sometimes described as "primitive," European anthropological interpretations of African culture helped reinforce white supremacist ideology.[28] Throughout enslavement, the white ruling class forced African spiritual traditions underground. Laws that prohibited drumming and gathering paired with the forced conversion of enslaved Africans to Christianity not only stigmatized African practices but also made them illegal. Misrepresentations of ATRs and ADRs as demonic persist within popular culture. Following the 2010 earthquake in Haiti, televangelist Pat Robertson falsely claimed that the earthquake was caused by the Bois Caïman ceremony that kicked off the Haitian Revolution, stating that Haitians "got together and swore a pact to the devil" to gain their freedom.[29]

Though ATRs and ADRs have been historically demonized, many of the core concepts and practices in African spiritual traditions are seen in a variety of different religions and spiritual traditions. Ancestor veneration, animal sacrifice, and nature-based rituals can be found in Indigenous American, Eastern, and Abrahamic religions. In recent decades, larger cultural interest in Eastern spirituality and European witchcraft has opened the door for ATRs and ADRs to grow in popularity. As the stigma associated with African spirituality lifts, more people are openly engaging in spiritual practices that incorporate elements of ATRs and ADRs. Interest in various spiritual traditions has grown among Black Americans seeking alternatives to Christianity and pathways to connect to ATRs and ADRs, even if indirectly. These traditions mix and meld spiritual practices from across and along the diaspora and offer another way for Black Americans to reclaim cultural connection. With this blending, practitioners are continuing to erode the stigma against practicing ATRs.

The Black witch movement refers to the exodus of Black Americans from the church in favor of spiritual practices rooted in African traditions, plant medicine, and divination. Modern Black witches incorporate a variety of practices, often drawing from traditions from across the diaspora while incorporating elements of astrology, tarot, and Eastern spirituality into their practice. The draw to Black spiritual traditions is especially strong among Black women and queer folks who have historically been marginalized by the Christian church. The ability for customization in modern Black witchcraft encourages practitioners to take what works for them and leave what doesn't, forming a complex culture based on inclusivity and tradition. Embracing alternative spiritual traditions rooted in African practices taps into the long history of Black spiritual resistance and liberation. As more people dive into these practices, many are realizing the hidden rituals and traditions already present within their own families.

African American and Caribbean practitioners are seeking out connections to their cultural practices and the spiritual traditions of their ancestors. Aborisa Porsche Little (@theorishasbaby on Instagram) sought out Lukumi and Ifá as a way to connect to her ancestral traditions that existed prior to enslavement. In a *Vox* interview, Porsche talks about the power in reclaiming traditions that connect back to her heritage. Porsche encourages curious spiritualists to question why the traditions that African and Indigenous peoples practiced were demonized by the church, an institution associated with colonization, enslavement, homophobia, and other forms of violence.[30] For many practitioners, the Black witch movement provides a safe haven for queer folks who have felt ostracized by the church to engage in a spiritual tradition that speaks to them. The ability to create your own traditions free from doctrine and dogma speaks to queer identity in a way that many organized religions don't. Through resources and witches on social media, more Black people are finding digital communities to learn more about ATRs and ADRs and other alternative forms of spirituality. Podcast host Juju Bae's *A Little Juju Podcast* serves as a conversational medium for spiritual exploration. Juju speaks about her own journey with spirituality as a queer hoodoo practitioner and iyanifa while interviewing different people who practice a wide variety of ATRs and ADRs. Juju talks about a range of topics that include the historical roots of hoodoo, the representation of Black witches in popular culture, and the struggle of communicating with chatty ancestors.

Bri Luna, most recognizable by her Instagram handle @thehoodwitch, was the first Black witch I stumbled across on social media. Back in 2016, her page, filled with crystals, tarot, and acrylic nails, caught my eye. Bri represents the modern Black witch movement in the ways she mixes astrology, witchcraft, and Afro-Indigenous practices. Incorporating a variety of traditions that combine her African American and Indigenous Mexican heritage, Bri blends modern and traditional rituals into a practice uniquely her own. In *Blood Sex Magic*, Bri recounts stories about the ways her grandmothers maintained familial traditions and passed down spiritual wisdom. She speaks about the fierceness and sense of independence instilled in her by her grandmother Sylvia. Although Sylvia had a difficult life, she passed down her pride in her Mexican heritage along with important life lessons. Her resilience and strength exuded a goddess-like energy that Bri reveres and embodies. Bri's grandmother Althea maintained connections to her hoodoo roots through food, healing, and cautionary advice. Bri remembers her grandmother's ritual of cooking collard greens on New Year's for prosperity and her warnings against leaving shoes around for fear that someone would "hot-foot you."[31] The spiritual teachings from both grandmothers play a major role in Bri's spiritual practice. Centered on divine femininity, Bri's incorporation of astrology, hoodoo, and Santería have earned her international recognition. *Blood Sex Magic* is the culmination of her lifelong practice, leaving readers with spells and rituals including limpia con huevo, instructions for making redbrick dust powder, and how to use tarot to catch a cheater.

CONCLUSION

There's a type of victory that lies in reconnection with ancestral traditions. In the face of white supremacy and colonization, being able to reclaim spiritual traditions and the tradition of resistance is a testament to the centuries-long dedication and determination of Black people. It's nothing short of a miracle to be able to speak to living elders, connect with digital communities, and read books that bring us closer to understanding our past so that we're able to shape our future.

The world we wish to create will look different than the world of our ancestors. We're navigating a political, environmental, and technological reality unlike anything humans have encountered before. We can learn from modern Black witches and incorporate elements from across the diaspora to create new strategies for survival in our rapidly changing world. By learning from our past we are able to shape and inform our future.

History reminds us that victory is not won in a single battle. It will take many victories, both big and small, to create a world grounded in the wisdom of our ancestors, free from white supremacy and capitalism. Victory begins with us, on an individual level. Before we can shape the world around us, we have to do the work to reshape our inner world. Our orí represents the personal divinity that lives within each of us. The most important relationship of our lives is the relationship we have with ourselves. Worshipping your orí can take the form of prayer or ritual. It also looks like developing a sense of integrity and intentionality within yourself and holding ourselves accountable when necessary.

The work of the Black Panthers reminds us that creating new worlds begins now. Rather than wait for the revolutionary collapse of capitalism and white supremacy, we have to begin building and transforming the relationships we have in the present. Through shared struggle, we can begin to imagine new ways of relating as we grapple with different strategies and ideologies on our path toward liberation.

CONCLUSION

I embrace the world! I am the world! . . . The essence of the world was my property. Between the world and me there was a relation of coexistence. I had rediscovered the primordial One.

—FRANTZ FANON, *BLACK SKIN, WHITE MASKS*

All that you touch You Change. All that you Change Changes you. The only lasting truth is Change. God is Change.

—OCTAVIA BUTLER, *PARABLE OF THE SOWER*

African traditional religions are not relics of the past. They are alive and in the process of evolving to meet the demands of Black people in the twenty-first century. Throughout history, Black people transformed and reimagined religion and spirituality, adapting traditional concepts and cultural expression to their contextual environment.

The structure of African traditional religions has shifted and changed over time, both shaping and being shaped by ADRs. From the spiritual practices of West Africa, a multitude of new spiritual traditions took root in the Americas. While these traditions retained many of the rituals, languages, and cosmologies of their African ancestors, they took on a flavor of their own, becoming something uniquely Black and uniquely diasporan.

For much of my life, I felt unanchored and disconnected from my ancestors. I couldn't see the ways my family fit into the tapestry of Black and African life across the diaspora. My family's story was told to me in bits and pieces, and it took me years to see the full picture. Although I don't know everything about my family, I've been able to put together the fragments of stories told to me by my parents and grandparents and weave them into the larger context of the African diaspora. My family's history and traditions have deep roots, stretching back across the Atlantic to the West and West-Central African coast.

So much has changed since my ancestors were taken from the shores of Nigeria and Kongo and brought to the Americas. There's no recourse for the violence of the transatlantic slave trade. Retracing our roots brings us closer to ourselves but it does not transport us back to the past. As African diasporans, our identities have been forever changed. In many ways our birthplace is the Atlantic, where both our gods and ourselves were reborn. In West Africa, there are common myths about why Africans in the diaspora have forgotten where they come from. Throughout history, enslavers attempted to eradicate the memories of the enslaved. Without stories to connect them to a homeland and history, they become easier to manipulate and control. Myths about zombies, trees of forgetfulness, and sorcery speak about the ways enslaved Africans were "tricked" into forgetting their past.[1]

The mass amnesia caused by the transatlantic slave trade is a myth. Despite attempts to strip us of our humanity and sever the bonds between mother and child, we always found our way back to ourselves. We didn't forget our past. We created a culture that reflects the rich history of our ancestry and honors the experiences we've had in the Americas. The wealth of our cultural heritage is felt through our food. We've created recipes inspired by African, Indigenous American, and European culinary techniques that nourish our communities. We've birthed new religions and spiritual traditions that combine wisdom from Yoruba, Igbo, and Kongo cosmologies with Christianity, tarot, and astrology to create diverse traditions that are personalized to our needs. We use tools from different spiritual practices to meet the needs of our present realities.

Through gender play, we've built a musical and cultural legacy that honors the diversity inherent within each of us. Stories about genderfluid orisas and genderless creators remind us that queerness exists all around us. Our ancestral practice of gender exploration lives on through the parties, balls, and performances that color Black queer life.

Urban farmers and herbalists are reshaping traditional agricultural practices and ancestral plant medicine, combining old techniques with new theories for survival. Through workshops, land trusts, and community gardens, Black people are reimagining ways to address food insecurity.

Growth is only possible if we look forward toward the future—and bring with us the tools of the past, like Ifá. Change is inevitable, and to face it we must learn to change with the world around us. Our greatest strength is our adaptability. Ifá is a flexible framework that can be applied and incorporated into preexisting ideologies. We can draw from different aspects of Ifá as we create new possibilities, grounding us in an ancestral understanding of the world while we look to the future.

GLOSSARY

aborisa A devotee of Ifá. Typically the title given to practitioners who have received their Hand of Ifá.

ADR African diasporic religion. The family of Africa-based spiritual traditions found throughout the Americas and the Caribbean, including but not limited to Candomblé, Santería, Lukumi, Palo Mayombe, hoodoo, Louisiana or Southern voodoo, Haitian Vodou, Winti, and Umbanda. ADRs are based on African traditional religions and can include varying degrees of Christianity and Catholicism, Indigenous American traditions and knowledge, Hinduism, and Buddhism.

agbo ilé The family compound.

àìkú Longevity.

Àjé The orisa of wealth.

ajogun Negative forces; see osogbo.

ATR African traditional religion. Indigenous spiritual traditions predominantly from West and West-Central Africa, including but not limited to Isese Ifá, Vodou, Igbo spiritual traditions, Kongolese spiritual traditions, and Dagara spiritual traditions. ATRs are typically associated with a particular tribe or ethnic group and consist of a wide variety of practices that have common themes of ancestral veneration and the veneration of the forces of nature.

aya Wife.

Aye   Earth.

baba   Father. Baba is also used as a sign of respect for elder men or leaders, regardless of whether they are fathers or not.

babalawo   Diviner.

ebo   Sacrifice.

egún   Ancestors.

ènìyàn   Human.

ẹsẹntaye   Yoruba naming ceremony for newborn babies.

Esu   The orisa of potential and possibility. Esu (also spelled Eshu) is called by many names in the diaspora including Elégbà, Elegua, and Papa Legba. He's associated with crossroads and is known for being a trickster.

Ibeji   The orisa of twins.

Ifá   Yoruba spiritual tradition. Also an alternative name for Ọ̀rúnmìlà, the orisa of wisdom and divination.

ikin   Sacred palm nuts used for divination.

iku   Death.

ire   Blessing.

irunmole   The primordial beings at the beginning of the universe. Ọ̀rúnmìlà, Esu, Ọṣun, Obatala are all irunmole. Irunmole played significant roles in creating the universe, earth, and humanity.

Isefa   Yoruba name for the Hand of Ifá. Refers to the process of receiving a personal Ifá shrine.

ìṣẹ́gun   Victory.

iya   Mother. Iya is also used as a sign of respect for elder women or leaders, regardless of whether they are mothers or not.

iyanifa   Translates to "wife of Ifá." The priestesses in the Yoruba tradition.

lwa   Haitian vodou spirit.

minkisi   Plural of nkisi (See nkisi).

mojo bag   Amulets made of clothes filled with herbs, crystals, or other spiritual objects for protection, luck, and healing. Also called gris-gris bags, mojo hands, or conjure bags.

nganga   Kikongo word for "priest." Nganga served as sacred healers in their communities, performing rituals for protection, healing, divination, and spiritual warfare. In Palo Mayombe, nganga also refers to the sacred cauldrons or pots containing spiritual energy.

nkisi   Ritual objects imbued with otherworldly power originating from Kongo. Plural minkisi.

obìnrin   Yoruba word for an anatomic female.

Odu   Both the orisa married to Ọ̀rúnmìlà and the sacred text of Ifá. During divination, symbols representing each odu are drawn on the opón ifá. The odu consist of oríkì, or sacred poetry. There are 16 major odu and 240 minor odu.

ọkọ   Yoruba word for the partner that is born into a particular lineage. Ọkọ has been inaccurately translated to "husband."

ọkùnrin   Yoruba word for an anatomic male.

omiero   Sacred herbal water used for healing and ritual cleansing.

ọmọ   Child.

ọmọ awo   Child of mysteries. The name given to new apprentices practicing Ifá.

opele   The sacred divination chain used by babalawos.

opón ifá   The sacred divination tray meant to represent the universe. Typically made of wood.

orí   The head.

orí-inú Inner head. Refers specifically to the spiritual head and personal orisa. Practitioners often worship their own orí. Special shrines are consecrated in honor of one's orí.

oríkì Yoruba spiritual poetry used during Ifá rituals to invoke the specific orisa or to manifest specific spiritual outcomes.

orisa The various manifestations of Olódùmarè, typically representing different aspects of nature and philosophical concepts. Orisas are often referred to as the "gods and goddesses" of Ifá and other ATRs and ADRs.

Orun Spiritual realm.

Òrúnmìlà The orisa of divination and wisdom. He is the central orisa in the ATRs and ADRs like Isese Ifá, Lukumi, Candomblé, and Santería.

osogbo Negative forces; also the name of a major city in Nigeria.

Ọṣun The orisa of fresh, sweet waters. Ọṣun is one of the primordial spiritual beings known as irunmole. She played a crucial role in the Yoruba creation myth and is associated with motherhood and freshwater.

Ọya Yoruba orisa of storms. Ọya is associated with the graveyard throughout the diaspora and is seen as the manifestation of transformative forces. She's known to wear a beard into battle alongside her partner, Ṣàngó.

Yoruba Ethnic group indigenous to Nigeria, Benin, and the surrounding region. The indigenous religion of the Yoruba people is Ifá.

NOTES

INTRODUCTION

1. Frank Baba Eyiogbe, *Babalawo: The Secrets of Afro-Cuban Ifá* (Woodbury, MN: Llewellyn, 2015).
2. Adérónkẹ́ Babájídé, "Elédùmarè/Olódùmarè (Olodum): Meaning, History and Significance: Sufficiency and Abundance," YouTube video, June 26, 2020, https://youtu.be/_CejQPUcDPg.
3. Dele Meiji, "Esu Is Not the Devil: How a Yoruba Deity Got Rebranded," *OkayAfrica*, December 14, 2017, www.okayafrica.com/yoruba-esu-is-not-the-devil.
4. Adérónkẹ́ Babájídé, "The Meaning of 'Ẹlẹ́gbà': The AfroLatinidad 'Eleggua/Legba,'" YouTube video, June 24, 2021, https://youtu.be/XEJWZYCo7pc.
5. Saidiya Hartman, *Wayward Lives, Beautiful Experiments: Intimate Histories of Social Upheaval* (New York: W. W. Norton, 2019), 42.
6. Malidoma Patrice Somé, *Of Water and the Spirit: Ritual, Magic, and Initiation in the Life of an African Shaman* (London: Penguin, 1995), 16.
7. William C. Anderson, *The Nation on No Map: Black Anarchism and Abolition* (Chico, CA: AK Press, 2021).
8. Baba Ifa Karade, *The Handbook of Yoruba Religious Concepts* (York Beach, ME: Weiser, 1994).

1. THE BLESSING OF IRE ÀÌKÚ

1. Adérónkẹ́ Babájídé, "In and of Itself 4: 'Egúngún' Is Not 'Masquerade,'" YouTube video, October 21, 2021, https://youtu.be/0up-uqxFeso.
2. Kimbwandende Kia Bunseki Fu-Kiau, *African Cosmology of the Bântu-Kôngo: Tying the Spiritual Knot: Principles of Life & Living*, 2nd ed. (Brooklyn, NY: Athelia Henrietta Press, 2001).

3. Jason R. Young, *Rituals of Resistance: African Atlantic Religion in Kongo and the Lowcountry South in the Era of Slavery* (Baton Rouge, LA: Louisiana State University Press, 2007).

4. Frank Baba Eyiogbe, *Babalawo: The Secrets of Afro-Cuban Ifá* (Woodbury, MN: Llewellyn, 2015).

5. Frank Baba Eyiogbe, *Babalawo,* 138–39.

6. Baba Ifa Karade, *The Handbook of Yoruba Religious Concepts* (York Beach, ME: Weiser, 1994).

7. Will Coleman and Awo Fa'lokun Fatunmbi, "Chapter 3: All of Creation Is inside of the Calabash," in *African Traditional Religions Textbook Ifá* (Pressbooks, 2021), https://pressbooks.pub/africanamericanreligionsifa/chapter/chapter-3-all-of-creation-is-inside-of-the-calabash.

8. Frank Baba Eyiogbe, *Babalawo,* 101.

9. Michael W. Twitty, "How Rice Shaped the American South," BBC News, March 8, 2021, www.bbc.com/travel/article/20210307-how-rice-shaped-the-american-south.

10. Michele E. Lee, *Working the Roots: Over 400 Years of Traditional African-American Healing* (Wadastick, 2017).

11. "The Gullah Geechee Herbal Gathering," www.gullahgeecheeherbalgathering.com.

12. Richard Evans Schultes, Albert Hofmann, and Christian Rätsch, *Plants of the Gods: Their Sacred, Healing, and Hallucinogenic Powers* (Rochester, VT: Healing Arts, 2001).

13. Richard Evans Schultes et al., *Plants of the Gods.*

14. Charlotte Resing, "Marijuana Legalization Is a Racial Justice Issue," ACLU News & Commentary, April 20, 2019, www.aclu.org/news/criminal-law-reform/marijuana-legalization-racial-justice-issue.

15. Black Bloom, "About," https://blackbloom.farm/Black-Bloom-Who.

16. "Declaration of Nyéléni," February 27, 2007, https://nyeleni.org/IMG/pdf/DeclNyeleni-en.pdf.

17. European Commission Directorate-General for Environment, "Field to Fork: Global Food Miles Generate Nearly 20% of All CO_2 Emissions from Food," European Commission, January 25, 2023, https://environment.ec.europa.eu/news/field-fork-global-food-miles-generate-nearly-20-all-co2-emissions-food-2023-01-25_en.

18. Leandro Pinto Júnior, "Sustaining the Traditional Production and Conservation of Creole Rice Seeds in Guinea-Bissau," Alliance for Food Sovereignty in Africa, 2019, https://afsafrica.org/sustaining-the-traditional-production-and-conservation-of-creole-rice-seeds-in-guinea-bissau.

19. Mulubrhan Balehegn Gebremikael, "Drought Tolerant *Ficus thonningii silvo-pastures* Sustain Livestock and Crops in Northern Ethiopia," Alliance for Food Sovereignty in Africa, March 2018, https://afsafrica.org/wp-content/uploads/2019/07/ficus-thonningi-eng-online.pdf.

20. John Yang, Kaisha Young, Juliet Fuisz, and Marconja Zor, "'Gaining Ground' Highlights Black Farmers' Efforts to Reclaim Lost Land," PBS News Weekend, July 23, 2023, www.pbs.org/newshour/show/gaining-ground-highlights-black-farmers-efforts-to-reclaim-lost-land.

21. Soul Fire Farm, www.soulfirefarm.org.

22. Leah Penniman, *Farming While Black: Soul Fire Farm's Practical Guide to Liberation on the Land* (White River Junction, VT: Chelsea Green, 2018).

23. Black Oregon Land Trust, www.blackoregonlandtrust.org.

24. "Residents Fighting to Save Compton Community Garden after Property Listed for Sale," KCAL News, May 2, 2023, www.cbsnews.com/losangeles/news/residents-fighting-to-save-compton-community-garden-after-property-listed-for-sale.

25. "Redefining Food Security and Community in Los Angeles: Urban Harvest: How Crop Swap LA Is Cultivating Community and Sustainability in the City," U.S. Fish & Wildlife Service, June 12, 2024, www.fws.gov/story/2024-06/redefining-food-security-and-community-los-angeles.

26. Apple Mandy, "Maya Feller's Rastafarian Ital Stew," BBC News, September 2, 2023, www.bbc.com/travel/article/20230901-maya-fellers-rastafarian-ital-stew.

27. Sarah Sax, "Finca Conciencia Is Building Food Sovereignty on Vieques Island," *Civil Eats,* May 15, 2019, https://civileats.com/2019/05/15/finca-conciencia-is-building-food-sovereignty-on-vieques-island.

28. Lakou Dantes, www.lakoudantes.com.

2. THE BLESSING OF ÀJÉ

1. Adérónkẹ́ Babájídé, "In and of Itself 2: Àjẹ́' Is Not 'Witch,'" YouTube video, June 6, 2021, https://youtu.be/Sv03NjVTO-0.

2. Walter Rodney, *How Europe Underdeveloped Africa* (London: Verso Books, 2018).

3. Emelyn Erickson and Louise Walter, "Law & Housing in Haiti," Haiti Lab, Franklin Humanities Institute, April 29, 2012, https://sites.duke.edu/lawandhousinginhaiti.

4. Aimé Césaire, *Discourse on Colonialism*, trans. Joan Pinkham (New York: Monthly Review Press, 2001).

5. William C. Anderson, *The Nation on No Map: Black Anarchism and Abolition* (Chico, CA: AK Press, 2021).

6. *Britannica*, "Africa," last updated December 14, 2024, www.britannica.com /place/Africa.

7. Saidiya Hartman, *Lose Your Mother: A Journey Along the Atlantic Slave Route* (Farrar, Straus and Giroux, 2007), 164.

8. Jason R. Young, *Rituals of Resistance: African Atlantic Religion in Kongo and the Lowcountry South in the Era of Slavery* (Baton Rouge, LA: Louisiana State University Press, 2007).

9. Saidiya Hartman, *Lose Your Mother,* 64.

10. Saidiya Hartman, *Lose Your Mother,* 63.

11. Saidiya Hartman, *Lose Your Mother,* 103.

12. Saidiya Hartman, *Lose Your Mother,* 104.

13. Frank Baba Eyiogbe, *Babalawo: The Secrets of Afro-Cuban Ifá* (Woodbury, MN: Llewellyn, 2015).

14. Frank Baba Eyiogbe, *Babalawo,* 16.

15. Judith Bettelheim, "Palo Monte Mayombe and Its Influence on Cuban Contemporary Art," *African Arts* 34, no. 2 (2001): 36, https://doi.org/10.2307 /3337912.

16. Judith Bettelheim, "Palo Monte Mayombe."

17. Jasmin Alejandrez-Prasad, "A Latina Bruja's Guide to an Egg Cleanse (Huevo Limpia)," *PS,* October 11, 2022, www.popsugar.com/smart-living/how-to -do-egg-cleanse-huevo-limpia-ritual-48963277.

18. Ina J. Fandrich, "Yorùbá Influences on Haitian Vodou and New Orleans Voodoo," *Journal of Black Studies* 37, no. 5 (May 2007): 775–91, https://doi .org/10.1177/0021934705280410.

19. Zora Neale Hurston, *Tell My Horse: Voodoo and Life in Haiti and Jamaica* (New York: Amistad, 1938), 138.

20. Gérard A. Ferère, "Haitian Voodoo: Its True Face," *Caribbean Quarterly* 24, no. 3–4 (1978): 37–47, https://doi.org/10.1080/00086495.1978.11829297.

21. Yvonne P. Chireau, *Black Magic: Religion and the African American Conjuring Tradition* (Berkeley, CA: University of California Press, 2003).

22. Yvonne P. Chireau, *Black Magic,* 77.

23. Yvonne P. Chireau, *Black Magic,* 126.

24. *Soul!,* season 1, episode 4, "Nikki Giovanni and James Baldwin in Conversation on 'SOUL!' (PART 1)," PBS, December 15, 1971, YouTube video, December 16, 2022, https://youtu.be/AFGkNEt30Fo.

25. W. E. B. Du Bois, ed., *The Negro Church: Report of a Social Study Made under the Direction of Atlanta University; Together with the Proceedings of the Eighth Conference for the Study of the Negro Problems, Held at Atlanta University, May 26th, 1903* (Atlanta: Atlanta University Press, 1903), https://docsouth .unc.edu/church/negrochurch/dubois.html.

26. Marilyn Mellowes, "The Black Church," PBS *American Experience*, n.d., accessed December 16, 2024, www.pbs.org/wgbh/americanexperience /features/godinamerica-black-church.

27. Jason R. Young, *Rituals of Resistance*, 43.

28. Margaret Thompson Drewal, *Yoruba Ritual: Performers, Play, Agency* (Bloomington, IN: Indiana University Press, 1992).

29. Zora Neale Hurston, *Tell My Horse*, 221.

30. Margaret Thompson Drewal, *Yoruba Ritual*, 184.

31. W. E. B. Du Bois, *The Souls of Black Folk: Essays and Sketches* (Chicago: A. C. McClurg, 1909), 189–91, www.gutenberg.org/files/408/408-h/408 -h.htm#chap10.

32. Jason R. Young, *Rituals of Resistance*, 93.

33. Tamara Williams, "Reviving Culture Through Ring Shout," *The Dancer -Citizen* 6 (May 15, 2018), https://dancercitizen.org/issue-6/tamara-williams.

34. Jason R. Young, *Rituals of Resistance*, 95.

35. Nick Montgomery and carla bergman, *Joyful Militancy: Building Thriving Resistance in Toxic Times* (Chico, CA: AK Press, 2017).

36. Charles E. Cobb Jr., *This Nonviolent Stuff'll Get You Killed: How Guns Made the Civil Rights Movement Possible* (Durham, NC: Duke University Press, 2014).

37. Charles E. Cobb Jr., *This Nonviolent Stuff'll Get You Killed*, 139.

38. Taylor Crumpton, "Why Do We Eat Black-Eyed Peas on New Years? Hoodoo," *Essence*, January 2, 2024, www.essence.com/culture/why-do-we -eat-black-eyed-peas-new-years-hoodoo.

39. Leah Penniman, *Farming While Black: Soul Fire Farm's Practical Guide to Liberation on the Land* (White River Junction, VT: Chelsea Green, 2018).

40. Andrew Lawler, "How the Chicken Built America," *New York Times*, November 25, 2014, www.nytimes.com/2014/11/26/opinion/how-the-chicken-built -america.html.

41. Vaughn Stafford Gray, "A Brief History of Jamaican Jerk," *Smithsonian Magazine*, December 22, 2020, www.smithsonianmag.com/arts-culture/brief -history-jamaican-jerk-180976597.

42. Leah Penniman, *Farming While Black*, 177.

43. Ralph P. Jean-Pierre, Amy D. Hagerman, and Karl M. Rich, "An Analysis of African Swine Fever Consequences on Rural Economies and Smallholder Swine Producers in Haiti," *Frontiers in Veterinary Science* 9 (October 12, 2022), https://doi.org/10.3389/fvets.2022.960344.

44. Leah Penniman, *Farming While Black,* 177.

45. Liliane Nérette Louis, *When Night Falls, Kric! Krac!: Haitian Folktales* (Englewood, CO: Libraries Unlimited, 1999).

46. "Barbados to Welcome Queen Quet of the Gullah/Geechee Nation," Queen Quet, March 19, 2019, www.queenquet.com/single-post/2019/03/19/barbados-to-welcome-queen-quet-of-the-gullahgeechee-nation.

47. Jessica B. Harris, *High on the Hog: A Culinary Journey from Africa to America* (New York: Bloomsbury, 2011).

48. Ayesha Harruna Attah, "Slow-Cooking History," *New York Times,* November 10, 2018, www.nytimes.com/2018/11/10/opinion/sunday/slow-cooking-history.html.

49. Bryant Terry, ed., *Black Food: Stories, Art, and Recipes from Across the African Diaspora* (New York: 4 Color Books, 2021).

3. THE BLESSING OF ỌKỌ/AYA

1. Oyèrónkẹ́ Oyěwùmí, *The Invention of Women: Making an African Sense of Western Gender Discourses* (Minneapolis: University of Minnesota Press, 1997).

2. Londa Schiebinger, *Nature's Body: Gender in the Making of Modern Science* (Boston: Beacon Press, 1993).

3. Londa Schiebinger, *Nature's Body,* 14.

4. Londa Schiebinger, *Nature's Body,* 17.

5. Londa Schiebinger, *Nature's Body,* 22.

6. Londa Schiebinger, *Nature's Body,* 25.

7. Londa Schiebinger, *Nature's Body,* 36.

8. Oyèrónkẹ́ Oyěwùmí, *The Invention of Women,* 12.

9. Oyèrónkẹ́ Oyěwùmí, *The Invention of Women,* 41.

10. Oyèrónkẹ́ Oyěwùmí, *The Invention of Women,* 33.

11. Oyèrónkẹ́ Oyěwùmí, *The Invention of Women,* 33.

12. Oyèrónkẹ́ Oyěwùmí, *The Invention of Women,* 38.

13. Ifi Amadiume, *Male Daughters, Female Husbands: Gender and Sex in an African Society* (London: Zed Books, 1987), 89–90.

14. Adérónké̩ Babájídé, "The Meaning of 'Ọ̀sun/Ọ̀ṣun': The AfroLatinidad 'Oshun/Ochún/Oxúm,'" YouTube video, December 5, 2021, https://youtu.be /sJ1a8OisWXA.

15. Mercedes Cros Sandoval, *Worldview, the Orichas, and Santería: Africa to Cuba and Beyond* (Gainesville, FL: University Press of Florida, 2006), 246.

16. Oyèrónké̩ Oyěwùmí, *The Invention of Women*, 45.

17. Oyèrónké̩ Oyěwùmí, *The Invention of Women*, 47.

18. Oyèrónké̩ Oyěwùmí, *The Invention of Women*, 55.

19. Saidiya Hartman, *Wayward Lives, Beautiful Experiments: Intimate Histories of Social Upheaval* (New York: W. W. Norton, 2019), 184.

20. Sabrina Strings, *Fearing the Black Body: The Racial Origins of Fat Phobia* (New York: New York University Press, 2019).

21. Saidiya Hartman, *Wayward Lives*, 189.

22. Saidiya Hartman, *Wayward Lives*, 338.

23. Saidiya Hartman, *Wayward Lives*, 308.

24. Adérónké̩ Babájídé, "AfroLatinidad Òrìṣà Song Translation 2: Bembe Oya Lafindae (Bè̩m̀bé̩ O̩ya La Fi Ń Dáa): Cuba," YouTube video, May 5, 2021, https://youtu.be/bv0DJV6bbGw.

25. Zora Neale Hurston, *Tell My Horse: Voodoo and Life in Haiti and Jamaica* (New York: Amistad, 1938), 221.

26. Margaret Thompson Drewal, *Yoruba Ritual: Performers, Play, Agency* (Bloomington, IN: Indiana University Press, 1992), 176–77.

27. Margaret Thompson Drewal, *Yoruba Ritual*, 176–77.

28. Zora Neale Hurston, *Tell My Horse*, 221.

29. C. Riley Snorton, *Black on Both Sides: A Racial History of Trans Identity* (Minneapolis: University of Minnesota Press, 2017), 57.

30. C. Riley Snorton, *Black on Both Sides*, 57.

31. C. Riley Snorton, *Black on Both Sides*, 60.

32. Saidiya Hartman, "Venus in Two Acts," *Small Axe* 12, no. 2 (June 1, 2008): 1–14, https://doi.org/10.1215/-12-2-1.

33. Saidiya Hartman, *Wayward Lives*, 284.

34. Chandler Owen, "The Cabaret as a Useful Social Institution," *The Messenger*, August 1922, 461, www.marxists.org/history/usa/pubs/messenger/08-aug -1922-mess-RIAZ.pdf.

35. Yale University Library, "We Are Everywhere: Lesbians in the Archive," 2023, https://onlineexhibits.library.yale.edu/s/we-are-everywhere/page /sapphic-blues.

36. Iván Román, "6 Key Figures of the Harlem Renaissance's Queer Scene," History.com, June 16, 2023, www.history.com/news/harlem-renaissance-figures-gay-lesbian.

37. Cari Shane, "The First Self-Proclaimed Drag Queen Was a Formerly Enslaved Man," *Smithsonian Magazine,* June 9, 2023, www.smithsonianmag.com/history/the-first-self-proclaimed-drag-queen-was-a-formerly-enslaved-man-180982311.

38. "Crystal LaBeija: The Queen Who Reinvented Ball Culture," PBS *American Masters,* September 24, 2021, www.pbs.org/wnet/americanmasters/crystal-labeija-the-queen-who-reinvented-ball-culture/18664.

39. Van Vogue Jam, "Ballroom Culture," accessed December 20, 2024, www.vanvoguejam.com/ballroom-history.

40. Julissa James, "Liberation Looks Like 500 Black People on a Dance Floor. Welcome to Hood Rave," *Los Angeles Times,* June 16, 2022, www.latimes.com/lifestyle/image/story/2022-06-16/hood-rave-l-a-black-queer-underground-party-dj-bae-bae-on-liberation-freedom.

41. Julissa James, "Liberation Looks Like 500 Black People on a Dance Floor."

42. Francisco Berreta, Sara Darehshori, Aisling Reidy, and Amy Branschweiger, "'I Have to Leave to Be Me': Discriminatory Laws Against LGBT People in the Eastern Caribbean," Human Rights Watch, March 21, 2018, www.hrw.org/report/2018/03/21/i-have-leave-be-me/discriminatory-laws-against-lgbt-people-eastern-caribbean.

43. Aditi Bhandari, "Uganda's Anti-Gay Bill Is the Latest and Worst to Target LGBTQ Africans," Reuters, April 7, 2023, www.reuters.com/graphics/UGANDA-LGBT/movakykrjva.

44. Enze Han and Joseph O'Mahoney, "The British Colonial Origins of Anti-Gay Laws," *Washington Post,* October 30, 2014, www.washingtonpost.com/news/monkey-cage/wp/2014/10/30/the-british-colonial-origins-of-anti-gay-laws.

45. Caleb Okereke, "How U.S. Evangelicals Helped Homophobia Flourish in Africa," *Foreign Policy,* March 19, 2023, https://foreignpolicy.com/2023/03/19/africa-uganda-evangelicals-homophobia-antigay-bill.

46. Human Rights Campaign Foundation, "The Epidemic of Violence Against the Transgender & Gender-Expansive Community in the U.S.," HRC, November 2024, https://reports.hrc.org/an-epidemic-of-violence-2024.

47. Biju Belinky, "Batekoo Collective," *Dazed,* April 29, 2019, www.dazeddigital.com/projects/article/44174/1/batekoo-collective-biography-dazed-100-2019-profile.

48. Bryant Terry, ed., *Black Food: Stories, Art, and Recipes from Across the African Diaspora* (New York: 4 Color Books, 2021), 209.

4. THE BLESSING OF ỌMỌ

1. Frantz Fanon, *Black Skin, White Masks* (New York: Grove, 1952), 127.

2. "Los Angeles Crowd Hears Islam Leader Ask End to Violence," *New York Times,* February 4, 1990, www.nytimes.com/1990/02/04/us/los-angeles -crowd-hears-islam-leader-ask-end-to-violence.html.

3. Adérónkẹ́ Babájídé, "In and of Itself 11: 'Ọmọ' Is Not 'Child,'" YouTube video, May 19, 2022, https://youtu.be/bGfuRY2ieoU.

4. Margaret Thompson Drewal, *Yoruba Ritual: Performers, Play, Agency* (Bloom-ington, IN: Indiana University Press, 1992), 52.

5. Will Coleman and Awo Fa'lokun Fatunmbi, "Chapter 3: All of Creation Is Inside of the Calabash," in *African Traditional Religions Textbook Ifá* (Press-books, 2021), https://pressbooks.pub/africanamericanreligionsifa/chapter /chapter-3-all-of-creation-is-inside-of-the-calabash.

6. Margaret Thompson Drewal, *Yoruba Ritual,* 54.

7. Akwaeke Emezi, *The Death of Vivek Oji* (New York: Riverhead, 2021).

8. Peter MacJob and Alex Last, "Nigeria, Twins and a Love-Hate Relationship," BBC News, May 8, 2024, www.bbc.com/news/world-africa-68977986.

9. "What Is a Doula?" DONA International, n.d., accessed January 13, 2025, www.dona.org/what-is-a-doula-2.

10. Donna L. Hoyert, "Maternal Mortality Rates in the United States, 2022," National Center for Health Statistics, Centers for Disease Control and Pre-vention, May 2, 2024, www.cdc.gov/nchs/data/hestat/maternal-mortality /2022/maternal-mortality-rates-2022.htm; "Disparities and Resilience among American Indian and Alaska Native People Who Are Pregnant or Postpartum," Centers for Disease Control and Prevention, May 15, 2024, www.cdc.gov/hearher/aian/disparities.html.

11. Alexis Robles-Fradet and Mara Greenwald, "Doula Care Improves Health Outcomes, Reduces Racial Disparities and Cuts Cost," National Health Law Program, August 8, 2022, https://healthlaw.org/doula-care-improves-health -outcomes-reduces-racial-disparities-and-cuts-cost.

12. Anika Nayak, "The History That Explains Today's Shortage of Black Mid-wives," *Time,* February 29, 2024, https://time.com/6727306/black-midwife -shortage-history.

13. Ifi Amadiume, *Male Daughters, Female Husbands: Gender and Sex in an African Society* (London: Zed Books, 1987), 74.

14. Pamela J. Brink, "Traditional Birth Attendants Among the Annang of Nige-ria," *Social Science & Medicine* 16, no. 21 (January 1982): 1883–92, https://doi .org/10.1016/0277-9536(82)90449-x.

15. Margaret Thompson Drewal, *Yoruba Ritual*, 209.

16. Margaret Moran, "Emergency Department Pre-Viability Delivery of a Fetus En Caul," *Cureus* 14, no. 2 (2022): https://doi.org/10.7759/cureus .22338.

17. Oyèrónkẹ́ Oyěwùmí, *The Invention of Women: Making an African Sense of Western Gender Discourses* (Minneapolis: University of Minnesota Press, 1997), 54.

18. Oyèrónkẹ́ Oyěwùmí, *The Invention of Women*, 52.

19. Margaret Thompson Drewal, *Yoruba Ritual*, 188.

20. Oyèrónkẹ́ Oyěwùmí, *The Invention of Women*, 53–54.

21. Dorothy E. Roberts, *Killing the Black Body: Race, Reproduction, and the Meaning of Liberty* (New York: Random House, 1997), 13.

22. Roberts, *Killing the Black Body*, 24.

23. Saidiya Hartman, *Wayward Lives, Beautiful Experiments: Intimate Histories of Social Upheaval* (New York: W. W. Norton, 2019), 90.

24. Saidiya Hartman, *Wayward Lives*, 90.

25. Saidiya Hartman, *Wayward Lives*, 92.

26. Daniel Patrick Moynihan, *The Negro Family: The Case For National Action* (Office of Policy Planning and Research, United States Department of Labor, March 1965), www.blackpast.org/african-american-history/moynihan -report-1965.

27. Hortense J. Spillers, "Mama's Baby, Papa's Maybe: An American Grammar Book," *Diacritics* 17, no. 2 (1987): 64–81, www.jstor.org/stable/464747, www.mcgill.ca/english/files/english/spillers_mamas_baby.pdf.

28. Saidiya Hartman, *Wayward Lives*, 94.

29. Roberts, *Killing the Black Body*, 41–42.

30. Roberts, *Killing the Black Body*, 36.

31. Roberts, *Killing the Black Body*, 35.

32. Roberts, *Killing the Black Body*, 43.

33. David Brooks, "The Nuclear Family Was a Mistake," *The Atlantic*, March 2020, www.theatlantic.com/magazine/archive/2020/03/the-nuclear-family -was-a-mistake/605536.

34. David Brooks, "The Nuclear Family Was a Mistake."

35. Daniel Patrick Moynihan, *The Negro Family*.

36. Nick Montgomery and carla bergman, *Joyful Militancy: Building Thriving Resistance in Toxic Times* (Chico, CA: AK Press, 2017), 98.

37. Sophie Lewis, *Abolish the Family: A Manifesto for Care and Liberation* (New York: Verso, 2022).

38. bell hooks, *All About Love: New Visions* (New York: William Morrow, 2001).

39. Stacey Patton, "Stop Beating Black Children," *New York Times*, March 10, 2017, www.nytimes.com/2017/03/10/opinion/sunday/stop-beating-black -children.html.

40. bell hooks, *All About Love*.

41. Roberts, *Killing the Black Body*, 51–53.

42. Emelyn Erickson and Louise Walter, "Law & Housing in Haiti," Haiti Lab, Franklin Humanities Institute, April 29, 2012, https://sites.duke.edu /lawandhousinginhaiti.

43. Saidiya Hartman, *Wayward Lives*, 101.

44. Saidiya Hartman, *Wayward Lives*, 91, 227.

45. Nick Montgomery and carla bergman, *Joyful Militancy*, 83.

46. Federal Bureau of Prisons, "BOP Statistics: Inmate Race," January 11, 2025, www.bop.gov/about/statistics/statistics_inmate_race.jsp.

47. Ashley C. Ford, *Somebody's Daughter: A Memoir* (New York: Flatiron, 2021).

48. Andrew Billingsley, *Climbing Jacob's Ladder: The Enduring Legacy of African -American Families* (New York: Touchstone, 1992).

49. D'Vera Cohn, Juliana Menasce Horowitz, Rachel Minkin, Richard Fry, and Kiley Hurst, "1. The Demographics of Multigenerational Households," in *Financial Issues Top the List of Reasons U.S. Adults Live in Multigenerational Homes*, Pew Research Center, March 24, 2022, www.pewresearch.org/social-trends/2022 /03/24/the-demographics-of-multigenerational-households.

50. Nick Montgomery and carla bergman, *Joyful Militancy*, 101.

5. THE BLESSING OF ÌṢẸGUN

1. Yvonne P. Chireau, *Black Magic: Religion and the African American Conjuring Tradition* (Berkeley, CA: University of California Press, 2003), 77.

2. Mercedes Cros Sandoval, *Worldview, the Orichas, and Santería: Africa to Cuba and Beyond* (Gainesville, FL: University Press of Florida, 2006), 224.

3. Jason R. Young, *Rituals of Resistance: African Atlantic Religion in Kongo and the Lowcountry South in the Era of Slavery* (Baton Rouge, LA: Louisiana State University Press, 2007), 111.

4. Jason R. Young, *Rituals of Resistance*, 112.

5. Jason R. Young, *Rituals of Resistance*, 113.

6. Jason R. Young, *Rituals of Resistance*, 116.

7. Yvonne P. Chireau, *Black Magic*, 62.

8. Zora Neale Hurston, *Mules and Men* (New York: Amistad, 1935).

9. Zora Neale Hurston, *Mules and Men*, 198–201.

10. C. L. R. James, *The Black Jacobins: Toussaint L'Ouverture and the San Domingo Revolution*, 2nd ed. (New York: Vintage, 1963), 86.

11. C. L. R. James, *The Black Jacobins*, 87, 88.

12. Yvonne P. Chireau, *Black Magic*, 64.

13. Yvonne P. Chireau, *Black Magic*, 65.

14. Yvonne P. Chireau, *Black Magic*, 67.

15. Frantz Fanon, *Black Skin, White Masks* (New York: Grove, 1952), 9.

16. Fanon, *Black Skin, White Masks*, 9.

17. Eldridge Cleaver, *On the Ideology of the Black Panther Party* (Ministry of Information, Black Panther Party, 1970), 1, www.freedomarchives.org/Documents /Finder/Black%20Liberation%20Disk/Black%20Power!/SugahData/Books /Cleaver.S.pdf.

18. Cleaver, *On the Ideology of the Black Panther Party*, 3.

19. Cleaver, *On the Ideology of the Black Panther Party*, 5.

20. Cleaver, *On the Ideology of the Black Panther Party*, 7.

21. Joshua Bloom and Waldo E. Martin, *Black Against Empire: The History and Politics of the Black Panther Party* (Berkeley, CA: University of California Press, 2012), 25.

22. Cleaver, *On the Ideology of the Black Panther Party*, 13.

23. Stephen Shames and Bobby Seale, *Power to the People: The World of the Black Panthers* (New York: Abrams, 2016), 13, 79.

24. Nateya Taylor, "More Than a Fashion Statement: The Symbolism Behind the Black Panther Party Uniform," National Museum of African American History and Culture, September 16, 2022, https://nmaahc.si.edu/explore/stories /black-panther-party-uniform.

25. Shames and Seale, *Power to the People*, 42.

26. Shames and Seale, *Power to the People*, 47.

27. Precious Adesina, "The Birth of the Black Is Beautiful Movement," BBC News, August 3, 2020, www.bbc.com/culture/article/20200730-the-birth-of -the-black-is-beautiful-movement.

28. Jason R. Young, *Rituals of Resistance*, 105.

29. Nadege Green, "The Black Religion That's Been Maligned for Centuries," *The Atlantic*, June 29, 2022, www.theatlantic.com/culture/archive/2022/06/vodou -haiti-misunderstood-religion/661429.

30. Nylah Iqbal Muhammad, "How Some Black Americans Are Finding Solace in African Spirituality," *Vox*, July 31, 2020, www.vox.com/2020/7/31/21346686 /orisha-yoruba-african-spirituality-covid.

31. Bri Luna, *Blood Sex Magic: Everyday Magic for the Modern Mystic* (New York: HarperOne, 2023).

CONCLUSION

1. Saidiya Hartman, *Lose Your Mother: A Journey Along the Atlantic Slave Route* (Farrar, Straus and Giroux, 2007), 155.

INDEX

ACKNOWLEDGMENTS

I'm incredibly grateful to all the people who helped me along this journey of writing my first book. First and foremost, I would like to express my deepest gratitude to my partner, Tobias. Tobias's love has supported me through every academic endeavor and throughout my journey of self-exploration and understanding. I'm grateful to have someone as intelligent and loving as Tobias in my corner rooting for me every step of the way.

I also want to thank my late grandmother Ida Louise and my late grandfather Johnny. Their love and presence in my life shaped my childhood and inspired me to learn more about the cultural context of their upbringing. My childhood memories spent in their Los Angeles home filled me with my earliest memories of the city I now call home. Not a day goes by that I don't miss them.

I want to thank my brother Gavin for our lifelong friendship that continues to grow stronger the older we get. I also want to thank my parents for encouraging me and being brave enough to grow with me on this lifelong journey. Because of you, I've continued to "keep my eyes on the prize."

I want to thank my best friends, Anita, Nkechi, and Paige, who are truly my sisters. I'm eternally grateful for our decade-long friendship and for our willingness to stand with each other through all of life's challenges.

This book would not be possible without the spiritual teachers and mentors who helped me along the way. I want to thank Chief Awósanmí Sékou Alájé, Iya Osuntoki, and 256 Healing Arts community for welcoming me into your ilé and guiding me along my spiritual journey.

Thank you to my editors Shayna Keyles and Margeaux Weston from North Atlantic Books for encouraging me and pushing me to be a better writer. Thank you for your patience, wisdom, and guidance throughout this process.

ABOUT THE AUTHOR

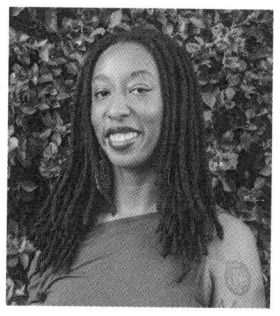 **GABRIELLE FELDER** (she, they) is a writer, data analyst, and aborisa born and raised in Orange County, California, and is currently based in Los Angeles. She received a BS in ecology and a BA in anthropology from the University of California, Santa Barbara; an MPH in environmental health from the University of Washington; and an MS in business analytics from the University of Southern California Marshall School of Business. Passionate about community work, she has trained as a postpartum doula, worked in community gardens, and led Afro-Indigenous ceremonies. Felder has shared her work through speaking engagements with the University of California, Davis, Women's Resources and Research Center and the Feminist Center for Creative Work.

ABOUT NORTH ATLANTIC BOOKS

North Atlantic Books (NAB) is an independent nonprofit publisher committed to a bold exploration of the relationships between mind, body, spirit, and nature. Founded in 1974, NAB aims to nurture a holistic view of the arts, sciences, humanities, and healing. To make a donation or to learn more about our books, authors, events, and newsletter, please visit www.northatlanticbooks.com.